The Ethical Foundations
of Social Work

The Ethical Foundations of Social Work

Annie Pullen-Sansfaçon
and
Stephen Cowden

PEARSON

Harlow, England • London • New York • Boston • San Francisco • Toronto • Sydney
Auckland • Singapore • Hong Kong • Tokyo • Seoul • Taipei • New Delhi
Cape Town • São Paulo • Mexico City • Madrid • Amsterdam • Munich • Paris • Milan

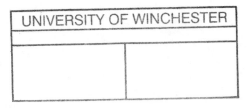

Pearson Education Limited
Edinburgh Gate
Harlow
Essex CM20 2JE
England

and Associated Companies throughout the world

Visit us on the World Wide Web at:
www.pearson.com/uk

First published 2012

ISBN 978-1-4082-2443-4

British Library Cataloguing-in-Publication Data
A catalogue record for this book is available from the British Library

Library of Congress Cataloging-in-Publication Data

Pullen-Sansfaçon, Annie.
  The ethical foundations of social work / Annie Pullen-Sansfaçon and Stephen Cowden. — 1st ed.
    p. cm.
  Includes bibliographical references and index.
  ISBN 978-1-4082-2443-4
  1. Social service—Moral and ethical aspects. I. Cowden, Stephen. II. Title.
  HV10.5.P85 2012
  174'.93613—dc23
                                                    2012001771

10 9 8 7 6 5 4 3 2 1
16   15   14   13   12

Typeset in *9.5/13pt ITC Stone Serif Std* by 32
Printed in Great Britain by Henry Ling Ltd., at the Dorset Press, Dorchester, Dorset

Dedication

Stephen: To Jacqui, who never lets the difficulty of the situation become a reason for losing faith.

Annie: To Dan and the children who make my life so complete.

Together we dedicate this book to all social workers who continue to keep alive the project of practical humanitarian social change.

Brief Contents

Contents

Preface

In 2006, the two of us began developing a year one module for social work students at Coventry University in the area of ethics and values. What we wanted to do was something that was both accessible and practice based, but which also sought to expose students to theoretical complexity. We felt this was necessary as much of the teaching we had encountered in this area tended to give students overly condensed versions of ethical theories with an over-reliance on the teaching of the existing codes of practice. While the latter certainly need to be taught, we felt that this approach needed to be turned on its head – in other words, that the starting point should be to teach ethical theories in their originary form. We felt that by explaining the way these emerged historically, what it was they were trying to address at the time they were originally articulated and how these debates developed over time, students and practitioners would be better equipped to use these ideas in practical situations. We also felt that this allowed students and practitioners to understand where our contemporary codes of practice came from. While there is no doubt that contemporary codes of practice are important and valuable within social work practice, they are in no sense a substitute for social work professionals who can think critically and independently. So rather than seeing codes of practice as the limit upon the horizon of debate in social work ethics, we wanted students and practitioners to see them as something which themselves were a product of a particular historical moment and which also needed to be critically examined and discussed. We wanted social workers to see ethical theories as ways of thinking through and around a problem, rather than as prescriptive guidelines. We also incorporated into our approach insights from sociology and social theory, again with a view to seeing these not as providing technical expertise or empirical justification, but as tools which sought to give students a better grasp of the complexities of moral concepts. It was on this basis that we developed a module based on this idea – that it is necessary to critically understand the ethical foundations of social work as a means of being equipped to apply those theories and concepts to everyday situations which were encountered in social work practice.

Of central importance within all this is the relationship between theory and practice; in particular, the capacity to understand the way situations in social work practice, as well as in life in general, represent practical embodiments of the concerns addressed by ethical theories. As a means of facilitating this within our module we used "Socratic dialogue" groups – a form of pedagogical activity which has been used to promote the development of practical reasoning.

The format for this would be that students working in small groups would address a question such as "Do you need to be a good person to be a good social worker?", but in answering this, they were only allowed to respond using personal experience. We then followed this up with a lecture looking at ethical theory, aiming to facilitate students grasping the relationship between the experiential and theoretical levels (see Pullen-Sansfaçon 2010 for a further discussion of this). Our students were very supportive of the way we had developed the module and this encouraged us further. However, one of the biggest challenges for this module was to find relevant and accessible reading to accompany our lectures. We found that generalist philosophy texts on one hand were a little dry and difficult for students to grasp, but on the other that the applied social work ethics books, while very practice-oriented, did not expose students to ethical theory and its application in practice in the way we were trying to. This book was written to solve this problem. Within this we have sought as much as possible to combine clarity with depth, promoting a theoretically rigorous approach to ethics, while at the same time making the material as accessible as possible for an undergraduate and postgraduate audience. Though the inspiration for this book came from very particular circumstances, we hope that the approach we have developed has a broader relevance to social work students and practitioners alike, but the extent to which this is true now resides with the question of how useful you, the reader, find it.

Stephen Cowden and Annie Pullen-Sansfaçon
Coventry and Montreal, 2012

Acknowledgements

As we note in our Introduction, the book began its life in the module "Principles of Social Work" which Stephen and Annie ran jointly with Level 1 students at Coventry University. We want to acknowledge the inspiration and encouragement we gained from our students in the way they responded to the ideas we developed. This module lives on as "Philosophy and Ethics of Social Work" and Stephen also wants to acknowledge the important role the students on this module have had in helping him develop his thinking in this area.

A number of other people helped us along the way and we would like to acknowledge them. Annie thanks Jeffrey Freedman for his proof reading of sections of the book, and Stephen acknowledges the helpful feedback he received from Gurnam Singh and John Woolham, who read and commented on various drafts. Our reviewers gave us invaluable encouragement at a time when we were not sure how this material was going to be received, and last but not least we thank the editorial and production teams for their enthusiasm in making this book happen.

Publisher's acknowledgements

The publishers would like to thank the anonymous panel of reviewers for their support with the development of the manuscript. The publishers would further like to thank the authors for the dedication, effort and skill they demonstrated in producing this book.

We are grateful to the following for permission to reproduce copyright material:

Photos

Page 9: Peter Higginbottam Collection/Mary Evans Picture Library; 14: © Chris Lawrence/Alamy Images; 106: Doug Savage (www.savagechickens.com); 139: © Pictorial Press Ltd/Alamy Images; 146: Jane Reed/Harvard University News Office; 148: © The Protected Art Archive/Alamy Images.

Every effort has been made to trace the copyright holders and we apologise in advance for any unintentional omissions. We would be pleased to insert the appropriate acknowledgement in any subsequent edition of this publication.

Introduction

We truly engage in ethics when we are not only concerned with our own freedom but also with that of others.

(Ricoeur 1990)

This book is concerned with introducing and examining a series of concepts which we see as making up what we have called the 'ethical foundations' of social work. These come from moral philosophy and from social theory, and we see the combination of these two as very valuable in exploring the kinds of ethical issues that are thrown up in social work practice. One of the key themes that we address throughout this book is that ethical practice never exists in a vacuum; it becomes real through the way practitioners use ethical concepts in concrete situations – and in a wider sense these situations are themselves located within particular societies in particular historical moments. It is in this sense that we see ethics as having a strongly social dimension, that is, they are concerned with the issue of how people relate to each other as well as how individuals and groups relate to social institutions. Many writers on social work ethics (such as Rhodes 1986, Clark 2006, Clifford and Burke 2009) have seen in this the political dimension of ethics, and we have also sought to develop this line of argument by drawing attention to the way ethical issues in social work are always contextualised and situated within power relationships. It is for this reason that 'conscious' ethical practice needs to be about questioning assumptions and critically challenging the various forms and structures of oppression which are encountered within social work practice.

This question of conscious ethical practice is a key theme throughout this book, and we have here drawn on the work of the contemporary moral philosopher Alasdair MacIntyre. In his book *Rational Dependent Animals* (1999) MacIntyre set out an argument for what he called the 'practical reasoner', and we see this idea as very useful for social work, and indeed something which may become an important paradigm for social work practice. MacIntyre suggests that people – in this case, social work students and practitioners – need to develop as practical reasoners. He characterises practical reason as a process which involves both reflection and self-knowledge; an enquiry that 'provides us with grounds for the criticism, revision, or even rejection of many of our judgements, our standards of judgement, our relationships and our institutions' (MacIntyre 1999: 157).

There are a number of reasons why practical reasoning skills are so applicable to social work practice. First, becoming a practical reasoner represents a set of understandings and skills which need to be consciously acquired and whose application needs to be worked on. It requires active engagement, rather than passivity, unquestioning reliance on external guidelines, or arbitrarily doing one thing in one instance and another elsewhere. Being a practical reasoner means developing your own voice, rather than just going along with what is happening around you because it has 'always been done like that'. Secondly, the concept of the practical reasoner situates ethics in a social and relational dimension. When we think of ethical dilemmas we often think of an isolated individual confronted by a series of difficult choices, but in reality the moral dilemmas that are dealt with in social work, if not in life in general, are invariably located in relationships with others as well as in particular institutional settings. In this sense ethical decisions are not simply individual decisions, but are decisions which involve other people, both directly and indirectly. This concerns the way questions about what people see as important are social questions. A key implication in this is the critical dimension of ethics, which is not just about an immediate situation, but is related to wider questions about what the role of a social worker is, and who they are meant to be accountable to–another key theme which runs throughout this book.

This concept of the social worker as practical reasoner is central to the way we conceive of ethical practice in this book, and we explore this concept in a range of different ways. Like other books on social work ethics, our approach is thematic, but the themes we have chosen take their starting point in theory and then work back to practice rather than the other way around, which is more typical. This approach has been adopted because we feel that a 'conscious ethical practitioner' needs to be able not only to grasp the realities of ethical dilemmas as they present, but also to understand the way ethical theories can help us to open up and better understand the issues within these dilemmas. As noted in the Preface, there is a tendency to approach the teaching of values and ethics primarily through the prism of contemporary codes of practice. While these are undoubtedly important, our approach has been to try to give students and practitioners an understanding of where these have come from, rather than seeing them as fixed and frozen – after all very few people would suggest that our current codes of practice will remain the same for even the next five years. An understanding of the development of moral philosophy is valuable for the way it allows us to see the relationship between the past and the present, and thereby understand the strength of the relevance these ideas continue to have for contemporary practice.

We have emphasised the importance of theory so far, but it is equally important to state that because ethics are a practice, they must bring together theoretical understandings with the acquisition of particular skills which are exercised in practice settings – it is in this way that practical reasoning skills are developed. It is therefore crucial that we locate the process of developing ethical consciousness within the real world of social work practice, and it is for this reason that we have made extensive use of case studies throughout the book. We draw from case studies not just to illustrate contemporary ethical dilemmas, but also to demonstrate the process of analysing the situation, making links between theory and practice, as well as applying a conscious ethical framework to a particular situation. The use of case studies allows the reader to conceptualise social work practice as a process in which ethical principles can be applied to concrete situations.

The book is presented in three parts, all of which include between two and three chapters each. The first part, entitled 'What is social work?', considers the historical evolution of social work up to and including contemporary policy perspectives. Rojek *et al.*'s pioneering investigation of social work's 'received ideas' (1988) made the important point that 'European Social Work can best face up to the actuality of value questions through a critical examination of its own historical roots and its received ideas in the context of their various discourses' (1988: 44). The first section seeks to recover the importance of this historic perspective as a means of revisiting the frequently asked question of what social work is. This work on social work's historical genesis is developed in the second chapter, which looks at the contemporary definition and manifestation of social work values and ethics.

Chapter 1 begins with the emergence of social work in the late nineteenth century as a moment in which the ethical boundaries of social work have been defined. We offer a comparison between two divergent conceptions of social work: the first and dominant tradition was that of the Charity Organisation Society (COS), which sought to reintegrate the 'outcast' poor into society through 'remoralisation', and then look by contrast at the Settlement Movement, whose focus was working alongside impoverished communities in partnership, seeking to develop the community's existing resources, as well as campaigning on issues of concern. By looking at these two traditions from which social work in its contemporary forms has evolved throughout the twentieth and twenty-first century, it is argued that social work has 'two souls'; one which emphasises the need for the socially disenfranchised to aspire toward 'respectability', and the other which takes as its starting point the real problems amongst people who are marginalised and excluded. The tension between these two conceptions of social work is then explored in a more recent period, in a discussion of the Radical social work movement in the 1970s and its critique of mainstream social work. We see the reconsideration of this period as important as it was also a moment in which questions about the role and purpose of social work were posed. While this movement was subsequently crushed under the weight of what Alex Callinicos has called the 'Reagan–Thatcher juggernaut' (2010: 8), we argue that there is still much that can be learned for contemporary practice by looking at the issues raised in this period.

Chapter 2 seeks to define the nature of ethics and values, looking at the meaning of these terms in the context of a number of ethical dilemmas from social work practice. Following Clark's (2000) argument, we question the conception of ethics as a *prescription* which dictates how to behave in problematic situations, and as a *discipline* that examines the foundations and the arguments on which the requirements are defined. The approach we argue for regarding social work ethics is one that takes into consideration the professional norms and standards in social work and also puts the concept of practical reason as central in the process of ethical deliberation. We also consider the social work value base as it is deployed within the current codes of ethics in social work, in particular within the International Federation of Social Work (IFSW) and the British Association of Social Work (BASW). Finally, we describe and illustrate some of the most common forms of ethical dilemmas in practice.

The second part of the book is entitled 'The social dimensions of social work ethics'. The chapters in this part develop the material raised in the first part with a focus on three key issues in social work: power, empowerment and bureaucracy, and their significance for conscious ethical practice. The chapters in this section work at the interface of social theory and ethics to consider the wider factors which frame the practical context in which social workers operate.

Chapter 3 begins by looking at the complexities of defining power within social work, and argues that the best way of understanding this is by looking at the way the term has acquired different meanings historically. We have then looked at ideas of power put forward by the philosophers of the European Enlightenment, the work of Karl Marx and Michel Foucault, as well as the importance of political struggles for class, gender and 'racial' equality. This chapter concludes with a case study in which the practical implications of these different ideas of power are explored.

Chapter 4 takes a more contemporary focus, looking at the trajectory of the term 'empowerment' as a concept which begins its life amongst community-based activist groups seeking a voice, but has subsequently become a key concept within the social policy universe of neo-liberalism. Why has this term empowerment become so important, not just within social work, but in contemporary policy and political rhetoric across the board? This chapter offers a critique of the way the term has come to be understood in such an individualised manner and offers some thoughts on how the term might be reclaimed for more progressive use in social work practice.

As we have discussed throughout this introduction, ethical issues within social work are invariably situated within organisational and institutional settings. This insight is particularly pertinent to Chapter 5 which looks at what a bureaucracy is and the different ways in which conscious ethical practice can be conceptualised within organisations. Are social workers always prisoners of the 'Iron Cage' of bureaucracy or are there ways in which we can exercise agency within them? We conclude this chapter with a discussion of managerialism and the impact that this has had on social work.

The third and final part, 'Theorising ethical practice', examines three core principles of social work through a number of ethical theories. We have chosen to explore three specific families of ethical theories which we believed have greatly influenced professional ethics in social work. We have done this because we believe that developing practical reasoning skills should involve a broad understanding and a critical appraisal of key ethical theories and their application to social work practice situations. Chapter 6 begins the exploration of social work's underlying roots in the moral philosophy of the Enlightenment. This chapter looks at the central concepts of self-determination and human dignity through the work of Immanuel Kant. The chapter will outline the way in which Kant's work has framed the understanding of these concepts in modern social work.

Social justice is another of the core values of social work which appears as such in the IFSW and BASW Codes of Ethics, and which, along with human dignity, serves as a central motivation and justification for social work action (IFSW 2000). Chapter 7 therefore explores this theme through a discussion of the Utilitarian theory of ethics from the perspectives of John Stuart Mill, and from the theory of justice as articulated by John Rawls.

The concept of professionalism is central to social work practice as deployed in the wide range of different ethical codes. Chapter 8 outlines that social work's professionalism can be understood to be based on the demonstration of different personal qualities that social workers are expected to embody in their work. It is through this theme that we examine a third position within moral philosophy which enables the contextualisation of the personal qualities and the importance of relationships between social workers and service users. The framework through which this is considered is through the work on relationship based and virtue ethics. The work of Aristotle and of contemporary moral philosopher Alasdair MacIntyre, who was mentioned earlier in this introduction, are explored, alongside debates on the ethics of care, an influential development of Virtue Ethics.

We conclude with a discussion of the centrality of ethical practice to social work as a whole, which expresses our hope that in writing this book we have made a contribution to keeping alive the concept of social work as a project of practical humanitarian social change.

Part 1

WHAT IS SOCIAL WORK?

CHAPTER 1

Social work histories

Chapter outline

In this chapter we will:

- Begin by considering some different definitions of social work
- Think about the reasons for this in terms of understanding the different trends within social work
- Seek to understand the way these have developed historically, seeing the different social and political forces that have influenced social work
- Focus on two historic periods – the 1890s and 1970s – as illustrations of the different ways in which ideas about what ethical practice in social work means have been manifested

The past, the present and the future are really one: they are today.

Attributed to Harriet Beecher Stowe
(1811–1896)

Introduction

When we talk about social work, what are we talking about? One of the complications of defining the nature and content of social work practice is that what it is varies considerably according to where it takes place. Sarah Banks has noted that:

> Social work has always been a difficult occupation to define because it has embraced work in a number of different sectors (public, private, independent, voluntary), a multiplicity of different settings (residential homes, area offices, community development projects), with workers taking on a range of different tasks (caring, controlling, empowering, campaigning, assessing, managing) for a variety of different purposes (redistribution of resources to those in need, social control and rehabilitation of the deviant, prevention or reduction of social problems; Banks 2006: 1).

There are social workers employed by Social Services Departments, those who work in national voluntary organisations for children, and others who work in small, grass roots organisations with homeless people. Are they all doing social work? Can they all call themselves social workers? Can we define social work independently of its context of practice? Just as the question of what activities actually count as social work has never had different kinds of answers, so equally we find different definitions of what social work is. Consider for example the following definitions:

Social work is 'a profession which promotes social change, problem solving in human relationships and the empowerment and liberation of people to enhance well-being . . . Principles of Human Rights and social justice are fundamental to social work' (The International Federation of Social Work [IFSW] quoted in Horner 2003: 2).

Social work is 'a very practical job. It is about protecting people and changing their lives, not about being able to give a fluent and theoretical explanation about why they got into difficulties in the first place' (Jacqui Smith, former UK Minister of Social Care, quoted in Horner 2003: 2).

When we think about these two definitions it becomes apparent that their authors are emphasising quite different conceptions of social work. The first definition, from the International Federation of Social Work, evokes a concept of the social worker as the agent of individual and social change, placing their skills at the service of the excluded and disempowered. While this definition sounds very positive and democratic, how much like the real world of social work do you think it is? The second definition from Jacqui Smith, former UK Minister for Social Care, by contrast, does not talk about social change, empowerment or liberation – instead it emphasises that social workers need to be 'practical'. This definition promotes the idea that social workers should be 'doers' rather than 'theoreticians'. At first glance that may sound a lot more realistic, but then we need to ask ourselves, if we are to practice ethically, don't we need to be 'thinkers' as well as 'doers'? Isn't there a danger in putting emphasis so much on doing that we fail to ask the question of what it is we are supposed to be doing? These are the sorts of questions we will be addressing throughout the chapters of this book, but the key point which will be explored in this chapter is that these different definitions are not just about people being confused about what social work is – rather this situation comes about because people's ideas are based on different assumptions about the role of social workers, which are themselves a result of different assumptions about society in general. Are social workers advocates and campaigners against injustice, or is their role simply to be putting together 'care packages' as quickly and efficiently as possible? Who are social workers supposed to serve – the organisations they work for or the service users they work with? Is the wider purpose of social work to serve the nation or to serve the citizen? In this chapter, we have approached this question by looking at the emergence of social work historically. We have done this because it enables us to see that social work never was and probably never will be just one thing – but that there have always been different and even radically opposed conceptions of the role and purpose of social work.

Social work ethics in history

Philanthropy, which means the process of helping others without expectation of personal gain, is as old as human society itself. Almost all societies have to deal with the fact that there are problems which manifest themselves on an ongoing basis and which will simply become more and more serious if some kind of help, assistance or relief is not provided. In his study of the origins of social work, Malcolm Payne noted that dating back to Ancient Greece and Rome there were important traditions of charity and philanthropy; these emerged from the need to deal with their own social problems, such as divorce, child abuse, abortion and prostitution (Payne 2005: 13). In medieval Europe, as well as in China and India, organised religion was not only one of the most powerful forces in society, but it came to be a focus for charitable work because of the association between religious virtue and assisting the more vulnerable in the community. Throughout history, there have been people who became involved in charitable work and set up organisations which sought to help individuals in difficulty. However, while the motivation to practice social work today may derive from these same underlying concerns for vulnerable others, social work as a structured profession existing within the contemporary welfare state has a more limited history, and it is this which is the focus of this chapter. As a formal profession, social work only came to exist in a small number of Western countries in the latter half of the twentieth century; it was not recognised formally in Britain until after the setting up of the welfare state and National Health Service after the Second World War. In terms of understanding social work's origins it is therefore important to understand the specific context in which social work as a profession emerged, and in which social work-type activities came to assume a certain importance and significance in a particular society. Social work as a profession therefore needs to be understood as something historically specific and which takes place within a particular context.

Before beginning to look at this history it is worth asking why a book on social work ethics might begin by talking about the need to have an understanding of the history of social work. The reason for this comes back to one of the key arguments we put forward in the introduction, which is that ethical practice in social work never exists in a vacuum: ethical choices are always grounded in a particular historical moment, a particular political period and a particular society. Take for example the issue of child labour. The vast majority of people who live in the economically developed world regard this practice as cruel and exploitative – they believe that children are too young for this type of work and that the right place for these children should be in school. Yet for many decades in Britain, children worked in mines, factories and farms. The rationale at the time was that poor families needed to have as many members of the family as possible working and bringing in an income: children just as much as adults were seen as capable of work. Employers themselves had absolutely no problem with the morality of child labour; as a campaigner against the practice noted in 1908:

> Child labour being regarded by the manufacturers as absolutely essential to the speedy piling up of fortunes, the morality of which no-one questioned, it was universally employed in the cotton mills and factories which sprang up in the land. Manchester, specifically the seat of the cotton trade from its earliest days, was a positive employer of child labour . . . A positive majority of the workers in the cotton mills were young children (Dale [1908] in Alexander 1988: 53).

It was only after major campaigns aimed at eradicating child labour throughout the early twentieth century, in addition to very significant changes in society in which attending school became to be seen much more important than working at this particular age, that child labour came to be seen as 'unethical'. In parts of sub-Saharan Africa and South Asia today child labour is practiced for much the same reasons as it was in Europe last century; poverty is widespread, there is little or no enforced regulation governing employment practices, and education is seen as the preserve of children from wealthy families. The key point here is that the very basis of what we regard as an ethical issue is specific to the kinds of assumptions and expectations people have of the way they will

Reflection break

Are ethical issues universal or relative?

One of the big debates in the field of ethics is the question of whether issues are universal, that is applicable in all situations, or relative, which means specific to particular contexts. In terms of this debate consider the following:

1 Child labour is now outlawed in most European countries, but does that mean that child labour was and is always wrong from the perspective of social justice? What is it about child labour that makes it morally objectionable?

2 Many religious organisations object to women who have unwanted pregnancies obtaining abortions on the basis that they consider this to be the 'taking of life', a major offence in the eyes of their religion. Consider a situation where group-based social housing for young people seeking to overcome drug problems is being provided by such a religious organisation. If the funding for this housing provision comes from the government, should the religious groups providing the housing be allowed to refuse to carry literature or information which gives young women advice about obtaining a termination? Would you consider the refusal to carry this information a legitimate expression of faith, or should the state, as funder, insist that women from all communities have access to information about the termination of a pregnancy if they require it? Finally, what are the mechanisms or principles we would use to decide on an issue like this?

live their lives. In that sense, ethical issues are always grounded in a particular context, so the value of having a historical understanding is that it allows us to look beyond our own immediate situation and values and situate those within a wider context.

This chapter does not offer a full history of social work from its origins until the present day, and readers who are interested in this may want to look at Malcolm Payne's 2005 book as a starting point for following this up. Instead we have chosen to focus on two key moments in the history of social work. These two – one from the 1890s and one from the 1970s – have been chosen because they were moments in which noticeably different conceptions of what social work was or should be came out into the open; what you might call struggles over the meaning of social work; what social work was *for* in a fundamental sense. We have chosen to focus on these two because they high-light not only the grounded but also the inherently political nature of ethical dilemmas in social work. This chapter begins with a discussion of the way social work in its current form emerged as a strategy for dealing with the con-sequences of social deprivation in urban capitalist societies, and then moves on to talk about the two historical moments. The first concerns the period of the 1890s where different ideas of what social work should be about emerged – the Charity Organisation Society (COS) and the Settlement Movement. These are both important for the way they influenced what became social work as an established profession within the welfare state. The second moment is con-cerned with the movement for Radical social work in the 1970s.

Social work as a 'product of modernity'

As already noted, the motivation which some people feel to help and assist those in distress is something which is universal to all societies, and probably to human existence itself. However, social work's arrival on the historical stage in the particular form which it now takes is a product of a particular history, and having a historical perspective allows us to grasp the way in which social

What is modernity?

Austen Harrington notes that the word modernity derives from the Latin word *modus*, meaning 'of our time'; here and now, as opposed to the past. It is this meaning that we evoke when we refer to something as 'very modern'.

However, the term can also be used to refer to a particular period, as we do here, where it refers to the influence of the Industrial Revolution, and the spread of the ideas from the French Revolution and the Age of Enlightenment (Harrington 2005: 17).

work's existence is related to the *emergence and persistence of particular kinds of social problems*. It is in this sense that social work can be thought of as a 'product of modernity'. We can think of modernity as a set of historical experiences based on capitalism as an economic system, industrial production, urbanisation and particular ideas about the political rights of citizens, which themselves emerged from the Enlightenment and the French Revolution in the eighteenth century.

Prior to the emergence of modern urban societies of the sort we now see across the economically developed world, the vast majority of the population survived through subsistence farming and people lived in small communities rather than in large cities. In medieval Europe people would not even have much of a sense of 'society', and Peter Knapp and Alan Spector argue that this idea is itself a feature of modernity. This is because what we think of as modern was defined in relation to the traditional subsistence economies which modernity was displacing. Hence it only became possible to 'conceive of "society" . . . when different kinds of social structure can be observed'. These different structures were represented by the conflict between 'two kinds of social system – one feudal, agrarian, monarchical, religious, aristocratic, traditional and rural, and the other capitalist, industrial, more democratic, secular, dynamic and urban' (Knapp and Spector 2011: 53). Karl Polanyi's book *The Great Transformation*, which traces the history of the emergence of capitalism in Europe, gives an interesting example of this. He demonstrates that the poor first became visible as a social problem in the sixteenth century as a consequence of the emergence of a group of people who were 'unattached to the manor "or any feudal superior"' (Polanyi 2001: 109). In other words, while the vast majority of people in medieval society lived in what we would consider today as grinding poverty, the problem of 'the poor' only came to be seen *as a problem* when groups of people who were not incorporated within traditional social bonds became noticeable.

For the development of capitalism to take place, first farming had to be industrialised, as it was through the introduction of machinery, and much land had to be enclosed. This meant the peasants who had for generations worked that land had to be removed from it, and this happened through brute force in many instances. It was through this process that a labour force for modern industry was created. What we call modernity thus arrived in people's lives through the destruction of centuries-old ways of life, as former peasants left the land, or were forcibly removed from it, and emigrated into new urban centres like the industrial British cities of London, Manchester and Birmingham. It is the momentous nature of these social changes which Karl Marx was seeking to understand when he wrote his now famous book *The Communist Manifesto*. He noted that:

> The bourgeoisie, wherever it has got the upper hand, has put an end to all feudal, patriarchal, idyllic relations. It has pitilessly torn asunder the motley feudal ties that bound man to his 'natural superiors', and has left remaining no other nexus between

man and man than naked self-interest, than callous 'cash payment' . . . All fixed, fast-frozen relations, with their train of ancient and venerable prejudices and opinions, are swept away, all new-formed ones become antiquated before they can ossify. All that is solid melts into air, all that is holy is profaned, and man is at last compelled to face with sober senses his real conditions of life, and his relations with his kind (Marx [1848] 1998: 6).

The key point Marx is making here is the way capitalism, a system he sees as driven by a new class of entrepreneurs he calls the bourgeoisie, needs to be understood as a radically different sort of economic system. In order to establish itself it had to destroy the feudal world and the 'ancient and venerable' social bonds associated with that, which brought about social dislocation, poverty and squalor on a scale never previously witnessed. As a commercial, and then an industrial society emerged throughout the eighteenth and nineteenth centuries in Britain, as Polyani puts it 'sporadic destitution had grown into a torrent of misery' (Polanyi 2001: 113). While the new factories producing goods that were now being sold across the British Empire created great wealth for this emerging class of factory owners, the vast majority of workers lived in unsanitary and impoverished conditions which were rife with disease and destitution. While rural communities had worked on a seasonal basis, the new factory work involved long hours and constant work. The older traditional communities had absorbed the disabled, the elderly and the frail within the structure of the

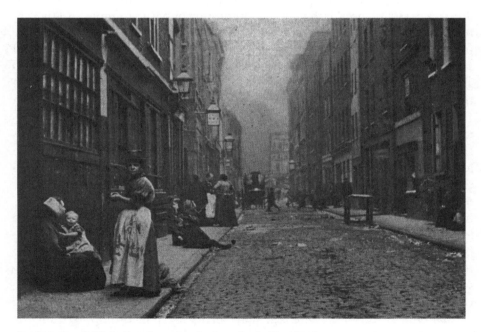

Back-to-back Victorian housing in London's East End
Source: Peter Higginbottom Collection/Mary Evans Picture Library

family; however, the need to care for those not able to work within the new system exacerbated problems of deprivation. We would argue that it was concern around the problems associated with the development of industrial urban capitalist societies that initiated the basis for modern social work.

Social work is presently a paid profession, and activities that we can think of as the forerunners of this emerged first as voluntary activities. Throughout the eighteenth and nineteenth centuries, a range of charities and philanthropic individuals expressed concern with the conditions of the poor. One of the most famous examples of this was a book put together by the campaigning journalist Henry Mayhew, which was published in 1851 with the title *London Labour and the London Poor*. In this book Mayhew and his team of researchers documented the impact which unemployment, substandard housing and rampant disease were having on the conditions of the working classes in London. The work of Charles Booth in the late 1900s developed this still further with the development of 'poverty maps', where social inequality indicators were mapped onto particular geographical areas.

While charity and philanthropic work were highly significant during the Victorian period, it would be a mistake to think the view taken by these individuals and groups was shared by the political establishment as a whole. The dominant view of political leaders and established opinion saw the problem as not so much concerned in terms of the suffering caused by poverty as the indolent behaviour of the poor – the frequency with which they engaged in drunkenness, 'idleness' and various other forms of 'vice'; in more strictly economic terms, 'unproductive labour' (Jones 1976). The poor thus presented to the governing classes both as an object of concern and as a threat, potential and actual, to the dominant order. This is significant for social work's emergence, because the justification for social work activities comes from both of these sources in different ways.

Many of the voluntary activities which were the forerunners of contemporary social work were forms of self-help which emerged from working-class communities themselves. Throughout the nineteenth century friendly societies, building societies and co-operatives, where working-class people pooled their resources to make payments during periods of sickness or unemployment, were formed (Payne: 33–4). These developments in working-class self-help were closely related to the growing influence of trade unions and the increasing belief that working-class organisations needed their own political party, which led to the founding of the Labour Party in the early years of the twentieth century. These forms of grass roots social work point to the way social work's legacy is linked to the history of socialism in places such as the United Kingdom, Australia and the United States (Payne 2005, Crocker 1992).

Charities, by contrast, were generally set up by philanthropists from the middle classes, often with religious motivations. The nineteenth century saw a substantial growth in charitable organisations, which were often set up within the major churches, but also partially separate from them. Typical of this was an organisation such as that set up by Thomas Barnardo, a mission preacher who had initially planned to work in China, but who, upon witnessing the destitution of orphaned and abandoned children in the East End of London, decided that his charitable energies were more needed in his own country. He set up a 'ragged school' in 1867 where children could obtain a basic education, and his first home for orphaned boys in 1870. Barnardo's entrepreneurial and fund-raising skills allowed this grow into a nationwide network, and the organisation he founded continues to this day (Payne 2005: 29–30). Middle-class women were also often prominently involved in organised charitable work, and one of the practices that developed out of this period was 'social visiting', where volunteers from charities would visit the houses of the poor, offering them advice on family life, budgeting etc. The origins of social work casework lie in this method of observation and recording (Jones 1998: 36). There were thus a range of different forms of provision which emerged with substantially different approaches – and this itself depended on the underlying philosophy of the organisation. This is significant because the different forms of provision which emerged in this period have all, in their different ways, fed into what social work as an organised profession became and is becoming. In terms of bringing this out we want to focus on two different organisations whose legacy to modern social work is fundamental in terms of the different ways in which they sought to provide assistance to the urban poor – these are the Charity Organisation Society and the Settlement Movement.

The Charity Organisation Society

The COS was founded in 1869 with the explicit aim of coordinating charitable giving. From the outset the organisation sought to provide key principles under which charitable giving was seen as desirable and beneficial. These principles were:

1 Full investigation into the circumstances of the applicant to be undertaken in every case.
2 No relief to be given that is not adequate, that cannot hope to render the person or family relieved self-supporting.
3 No relief to be given to cases that are so 'bad' in point of character or so chronic in their need as to be incapable of permanent restoration.
4 All 'hopeless' cases, however deserving, to be handed over to the poor law (Townsend [1911] in Alexander 1998: 183).

As the principles above imply, the COS model of welfare was based on the idea that the poor had to demonstrate particular qualities – such as patience, cleanliness, thrift, sobriety and in particular the ability to become 'self-supporting' – in order to be seen as worthy of receiving help. The family was assessed through the process of 'social visiting', where middle-class women volunteers would visit the houses of the poor, offering what was seen as appropriate advice, and most importantly assessing them for whether the family was deemed to be worthy or unworthy of receiving charity. The influential secretary of the organisation, Loch, argued that unless this process of assessing families was undertaken, charitable giving was 'as husks, flung before the poor as if they were without common humanity' (in Payne 2005: 35). This reflects the underlying fear within large sections of the political establishment that while charitable giving was worthy, there was also the danger that it would simply encourage dependency and idleness from key sections – particularly the unskilled – of the working classes.

As well as contributing the casework method and the model of home visiting to modern social work, the COS model instituted the process of allocating support based on a distinction between the 'deserving' and the 'undeserving'. Underlying this was an idea central to charitable social work; that its role lay in reforming the 'characters' of the poor. Bernard Bosanquet, a leading member of the COS, expressed this as follows:

> Here then we find the true meaning of social work. Whenever it may start its goal is the same; to bring the mind into order; into harmony with itself. Social disintegration is the outward and visible form of moral and intellectual disintegration (in Jones 1998: 36).

The COS approach was thus an individualist model which placed the responsibility on the applicant for charity to demonstrate they had the capacity to 'raise themselves up' beyond the difficulties caused by poverty, unemployment and destitution. This implies that difficulties experienced were essentially individual misfortunes rather than structural features of the wider society and economy, and the despair and demoralisation resulting from these were seen as moral failings, rather than responses to feelings of powerlessness and isolation.

While Bosanquet's sentiments may appear crude and patronising to contemporary ears, Chris Jones has argued that this conception of social work has had a profound influence:

> Despite the many changes in language and knowledge base of social work since the end of the nineteenth century, social work has remained an activity that is not only class specific, but has also continued to practice as if the primary causes of clients' problems are located in their own behaviour, morality and deficient family relationships. Mainstream social work, despite its immersion in poverty and amongst the least powerful sections of the population, has rarely ventured to seek explanations for these difficulties beyond family and interpersonal relationships and dynamics (Jones 1998: 37).

As well as raising questions about how social workers understand and make sense of the experiences of service users, Jones is also raising the question about how the organisational context of social work influences the ethical decision making which social workers undertake, an issue which will be picked up in Chapter 5 on bureaucracy. Jones' point is also significant because he is

Reflection break

How much do social workers acknowledge poverty as a factor in their assessments of service users?

There is considerable evidence to demonstrate the fact that contemporary children and families social work intervention is almost entirely experienced by the poorest and most socially marginalised families in society. Discuss the following questions:

1 Why do you think it is that the poverty is such a consistent factor in families seen by children and families social workers?

2 What impact might this have on the way these families experience social work intervention?

3 Are there things that social workers can do about this? What are they?

suggesting that the legacy of the COS model of social work is far more influential than is generally acknowledged.

The Settlement Movement

An altogether different vision of the role of social work in the late Victorian era was the Settlement Movement. Settlements were a significant social reform initiative which consisted of students and well-educated groups moving into deprived areas and using their skills to facilitate a greater level of education, dignity and quality of life for working-class communities. The original Settlement in the UK was Toynbee Hall in Whitechapel in East London, which was established by Canon Samuel Barnett in 1884. Clement Attlee, one of the architects of British welfare state, was closely involved in Toynbee Hall as a young man. There were other settlements across the UK and another very famous one, Hull House, in Chicago, in which the social reformer and feminist Jane Addams was a founding figure. In her autobiography Jane Addams describes an incident which was pivotal in demonstrating what was wrong with the charity model of social work, with its central distinction between the deserving and the undeserving, and which went on to shape the direction in which she took social work at Hull House Settlement. Describing her early involvement in charity work, she explains that she was given the task of assisting a man who had lost his job as a shipping clerk:

> I told him of an opportunity for work on the drainage canal and intimated that if any employment were available, he ought to exhaust that possibility before asking for help. The man replied that he had always worked indoors and that he could not endure outside work during the winter. I am grateful to remember that I was too uncertain to be severe, but that I held to my instructions. He did not come again

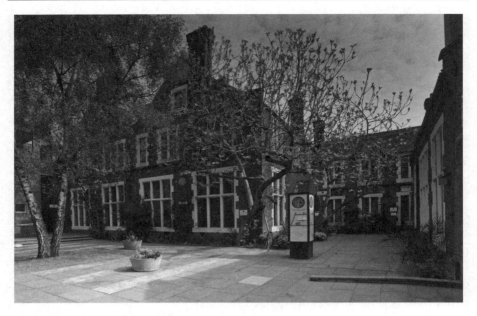

Toynbee Hall, in Whitechapel, London
Source: © Chris Lawrence/Alamy

for relief, but worked for two days on the canal, where he contracted pneumonia and died a week later. I have never lost trace of the two little children he left behind him, although I cannot see them without a bitter consciousness that it was at their expense I learned that life cannot be administered by definite rules and regulations; that wisdom to deal with a man's [sic] difficulties comes only through knowledge of his life and habits as a whole, and that to treat an isolated episode is almost sure to invite blundering (in Conway 1992: 518–19).

Settlements in this sense emerged out of a critique of the individualist nature of the dominant Victorian charity model. Beatrice Webb, a committed socialist who was involved in numerous disputes with Bernard Bosanquet of the COS in the UK, argued for the need to understand poverty as a structural problem, and it was this that was central to the philosophy of the Settlements.

While the Settlement Movement was, like most forms of nineteenth-century social work, inspired by Christianity, the philosophy of Settlements tended towards a more radical reading of the gospels than the COS and other church-based charities. As W. Moore Ede explains, the philosophy of the Settlements was not about conversion of those seen to be suffering from deficiencies of character. Those living in deprived areas:

Will not be converted by missionaries and tracts sent by dwellers in the West End. The dwellers in the West End must go to the dwellers in the East themselves, share with the East those pleasures which give interest and delight to the dwellers in the West, and make up the fullness of their lives (in Woodrofe 1962: 65).

Active participation in the lives of people living in deprived areas was therefore central to the ethos of the Settlement Movement, reflecting the idea that in order to change the degraded conditions in which communities were living, you needed to understand through first-hand experience the kinds of pressures and difficulties which they faced. Unlike the COS approach in which the individual was assessed according to strictly defined rules, the Settlement Movement involved a more collaborative relationship between helper and helped, emphasising the value of allowing the helper and the helped to learn from each other.

The two souls of social work

One of the great founders of the Social Sciences was a Frenchman named August Comte (1798–1813); he argued that one of the most important things that people in modern societies had to learn was the capacity for altruism – which he defined as 'living for others' (Dixon 2008). This kind of idea is crucial to the development of social work, and interestingly enough we can see it as something which animates and motivates both the Settlement Movement and the COS, as well as being an ethical concept which is still central to contemporary social work. However, while both conceptions of social work could agree on the value of 'living for others', the interpretations of what this meant were profoundly different. The COS volunteers and leaders certainly saw themselves as living for others, and they were motivated by concerns about the appalling conditions in which poor people lived in Britain's industrial cities. However, they did not question the dominant order, and saw the helping role of social work in terms of encouraging individuals facing difficulties to reform and change themselves so as to adapt and conform to the status quo. While the COS was a charitable organisation, one of its central concerns was that the poor needed to show their willingness to become self-supporting; that is, to go out to work. In this sense the COS shared the fears, which we have noted were dominant with the political establishment of the time, that charitable giving could potentially encourage idleness among the poor. Work was understood by the COS volunteers as an expression of religious virtue; by helping people to become self-supporting they were helping people to be 'better people'. What this leaves out of the picture is the experience described by Jane Addams – the unsafe, unsanitary and exploitative conditions in which work was frequently undertaken. In the sense in which they overlooked this, charities such as the COS could be seen as one of many social mechanisms which sought to discipline, cajole or enforce the working classes into involvement with what was seen as 'productive labour'. As Mrs Townsend, a Fabian critic of the COS, commented at the time:

> They stuck to the theory of individual independence . . . in a world where man-made laws were enabling the rich to grind the faces of the poor (Townsend [1911] in Alexander 1998: 184).

The Settlement Movement by contrast sought to work around practical problems from the perspective of, in the words of Jane Addams, 'knowledge of the lives and habits' of the community as a whole. Rather than seeing the problems of poverty and destitution as problems of individual character, they promoted a concept of social work based on campaigning, advocacy alongside practical measures to improve the lives of people. We see the two approaches to social problems embodied in these two movements as representing 'the two souls of social work': one representing a vision of social work based on the reform of individual character and support for the 'deserving poor', and the other representing an attempt to understand the circumstances of communities which experience poverty as a whole, and working alongside those communities in a collaborative manner. They also represent social work's two souls because the different assumptions and values embodied have both become incorporated into what social work became once it was formally institutionalised within the state. Social work's political legacy is therefore a contradictory one – and it is important to be aware of this in the context of social work ethics because the two approaches offer different ways of understanding and conceptualising the sorts of ethical issues thrown up in social work today. In concrete terms, how much in social work practice today do we see problems such as the neglect of children purely in terms of action, or inaction, by 'bad parents'? How much are problems like this related to the structure of society, and people marginalised from society through exclusion from the labour market and poverty? And if this is the case, what can be done in social work practice to incorporate recognition of this? These issues return us to the question of whom social work is supposed to serve – the individual, the community or the nation?

The emergence of state social work

As already noted, these two conceptions of social work derived from a time when social work was a voluntary activity, and governmental involvement in the arena of welfare provision was minimal. It was the experience of the Great Depression in the 1930s, followed by the Second World War, which substantially changed the political landscape, and in Britain brought about the election of a post-war Labour government which sought to institutionalise welfare within the state. This represented a major change and Richard Titmuss has argued that the essential precondition for this was that 'the circumstances of the war created an unprecedented sense of social solidarity among the British people, [and] made them willing to accept a great increase of egalitarian policies and collective state intervention' (in Thane 1982: 223).

At the level of policy it was the Beveridge Report in 1942 which acted as the founding document for development of the welfare state, proposing a blueprint for fighting against the five evils of the modern world: want, disease, ignorance, squalor and idleness. The report's solution to this was a free, universal and comprehensive provision of service from 'the cradle to the grave' in the spheres of both social care and health, with the creation of the National Health Service (Payne 2005). Following the election in 1945 of the Labour government led by Clement Attlee, which implemented these major changes, the welfare state slowly began to take shape in the form of a universal system, aimed at providing services to everyone in need of health and social assistance. It was during this period that social work came to be institutionalised as one of the key professions within the welfare state, and this change meant that social work moved from being a voluntary activity to a public service with legally defined roles and responsibilities. John Harris has characterised this as the period of what he has called 'the bureau-professional regime' in social work – meaning the professional as expert (Harris 1999). Throughout the subsequent decades of the 1950s, 1960s and 1970s in Britain the responsibilities of social workers grew and developed, extending into completely new areas such as mental health and juvenile delinquency. The framework of statutory responsibilities for social work also developed, encompassing such crucial issues such as childcare and mental health. The most significant reorganisation of social work took place in the wake of the Seebohm Report in 1968, which sought to rationalise and simplify access to services, leading to the development of Social Services Departments within Local Authorities. The report sought to recommended the creation of 'a new Local Authority department, providing a community based and family oriented service, which will be available to all' (Seebohm Report, cited in Harris 1999: 919). Harris notes that the Seebohm Report

> represented the consolidation of social work's position as part of the post-war social democratic welfare state . . . The period has been described as the 'high tide of social work' coming at the tail-end of the commitment of 1960s social democracy to tackling the problems of society through expertise located in the state and to promoting citizenship through solidarity (1999: 920).

Alongside the growth of social work provision in Local Authorities, social work education in colleges and universities also became formalised during the early 1960s. State-based social work was never intended to eliminate the need for voluntary activity, and this period also witnessed the growth of the 'voluntary sector', which was itself increasingly professionalised, though its name was a reminder of its earlier history. However, from this point onwards the vast majority of social work took place within Local Authorities.

Radical social work

While the institutionalisation of social work brought about extensive growth and development of the profession, many of the old questions about the role and allegiances of social work had not gone away – indeed with increasing amounts of statutory responsibilities they had begun to return in new ways. Just as the Seebohm Report sought to institutionalise and clarify the social work role still further, stirrings took place within social work which posed questions of whether the casework model, and the concurrent concept of professional expertise, could not be responsible for individualising and pathologising what were in fact social and structural problems. Harris has noted that while the Seebohm Report's conception of public service was strongly universalist:

> . . . what was missing . . . was a consideration of the authority dimension present in bureau-professional regimes or any explicit discussion of the rights service users might need to safeguard their position when faced with bureau-professional authority (1999: 920–1).

It could be seen to be this question of whom social work served, and of the basis of their professional role vis-à-vis the experiences of service users, which formed one of the central concerns which surfaced most visibly in the critique of social work developed by the Radical social work movement. Though this movement was small and short-lived, it has as Powell noted 'exercised an influence . . . totally out of proportion to its minority status' (2001: 68). This may be partial because its concerns were shared by many who were never actively involved in it, but also because it represented a critique of professional authority which was an important theme in the emergence of community activism during this period. In thinking about the origins and basis of the welfare state in post-war Britain, Gail Lewis has argued that the 'old' welfare state was never 'a single homogenous entity' but rather 'a series of overlapping and negotiated positions through which relations between a number of actors were articulated' (1998: 40). The key point Lewis was making here is that the post-war welfare state was based on a series of assumptions about entitlements which grew out of a particular period of history. It was in this period of social change accompanied by greater politicisation that many of these assumptions came to be questioned. An example of this is the concept of the 'family wage', where it was assumed that the male wage-earner was the primary breadwinner for the family, and the woman's role in the family was as a housewife or a subservient breadwinner. These patriarchal assumptions came to be challenged by a new generation of women who wanted to enter the workforce and the professions. Women in the trade union movement also fought a political battle to obtain equal pay for the same work as male workers, demanding that their work be recognised as of equal value, and it was this that played a key role in the development of equal pay legislation. Another example was the campaign waged by the black community in Britain concerning the disproportionate number of children from African-Caribbean backgrounds who were classified 'educationally subnormal', and placed in separate educational institutions, known popularly as 'sin-bins' (Coard 2005, CCCS 1982). This was significant because it was a community-based campaign which contested the idea of professional expertise being benign by pointing to the way that professional decisions, far from being enlightening, could be racist and discriminatory. It also concerned the demand by parents to have a say about what happened in schools, rather than this being determined solely by educational professionals. In this sense these struggles were paralleled by those of other groups of parents who questioned medical decisions to place groups, such as people with learning disabilities, in institutionalised care.

Radical social work can be seen as a response to this more politicised milieu in which it was believed that the social work role should be that which enabled service users to change their situation through collective action, rather than as the expert professional. The authors of the book *In and Against the State* (CSE 1980) expressed this as a generalised viewpoint when they argued that:

> It is not just that state provision is under-resourced, inadequate, and on the cheap. The way it is resourced and administered to us doesn't seem to reflect our real needs (1980: 9).

Radical social work wanted social work to be more grass roots and egalitarian, and sought to break down the professional distance between themselves and the communities who were the clients of social work. As Bailey and Brake argued in their book *Radical Social Work*:

> Radical social work is essentially understanding the position of the oppressed in the social and economic context they live in . . . Professionalism firstly implies the acquisition of a specialism – knowledge and skills not possessed by untrained workers. This isolates the social worker from the population at large. Secondly, social workers come to see themselves . . . on a par with doctors and lawyers. Thirdly, it encourages the introduction of businesslike career structures where 'correct' and 'professional' behaviour (such as detachment and controlled emotional involvement) is rewarded with advancement (1975: 145).

The title of the Radical Social Work magazine was *Case Con*, implying that casework's individualising 'professional knows best' assumption was an ideological smokescreen which prevented people from understanding the underlying causes of social problems. As the group wrote in their manifesto:

> One important tool of professional Social Work has been casework – a pseudo-science – that blames individual inadequacies for poverty and so mystifies and diverts attention from the real causes – slums, homelessness and economic exploitation. The casework ideology forces clients to be seen as needing to be changed to fit society. Professionalism is a particularly dangerous development specifically because social workers look to it for an answer to many of the problems and contradictions of the job itself – i.e. being unable to solve the basic inadequacy of society through social work. It must be fought at every opportunity (www.radical.org.uk/barefoot/casecon.htm).

Lavalette and Ferguson have identified two main foci of the groups. The group around *Case Con* emphasised:

> rank and file activism, the encouragement of democracy within the workplace and the union, and the development of closer links between workers and clients on the basis of common class interests. A second strand also described itself as Marxist and

similarly stressed the need for closer links between social workers, clients and trade unions but placed more emphasis on consciousness raising with clients on one hand, and on working within the official structures of the Labour Party and Trade Unions on the other (2007: 22).

These statements give a sense of the politics of Radical social work. While in a sense these arguments could be seen as a re-statement of the earlier arguments of the advocates of Settlements against the COS, the difference was that social work as a profession had gone on to become a significant grouping within the welfare state. Radical social work was thus an oppositional movement within the social work profession. While the arguments they made for a more egalitarian approach were important, it is also true that, as Yelloly commented, 'it was easier to see what Radical social work was against rather than what it was for in terms of alternative practice' (in Rojek *et al.* 1988: 46). Much of this revolves around the dilemmas of being 'in and against the state'. The Settlements developed in a period in which the state actively resisted involvement in social welfare, a position which the Settlement leaders argued against. Radical social work raised the same issues, but from the period where social work had successfully carved out a position for itself as one of the key professional groupings within the welfare state. One of the ways in which Radical social work dealt with this contradiction was to emphasise the need for social workers to be involved in trade unions; and while participation in unions was entirely consistent with their overall approach, it is not the same as an alternative social work practice. It is also the case that while particular kinds of social work, such as social workers who were involved in claimants unions or tenants associations, could see in their practice 'common class interests' between themselves and the people they were working with, it is not easy to see how this is the case for other forms of social work, such as child protection, for example. Indeed, it was scandals around child protection that were used by the incoming Conservative government of Margaret Thatcher to undermine the credibility of social work, and with that, the welfare state as a whole.

The problem for Radical social work lay in the way the context changed and the debate shifted radically from a situation where they were questioning the basis of social work, to a situation in which the profession as a whole was under attack from leading figures in the government, alongside a huge swathe of cuts in public expenditure and a series of unrelenting attacks on the trades unions. With the emergence of the New Right in Britain and the United States throughout the 1980s, a new common sense emerged regarding the detrimental impact of the state's involvement in social welfare. It is salutary to note that in making this argument, the New Right appropriated much of the antiprofessional rhetoric of radical movements, and this is a point we develop in Chapter 4, which discusses empowerment. Mary Langan has similarly noted that one of the great ironies of Radical social work was that while as a political movement it had died out by the mid-1980s, its language and rhetoric lived on; indeed 'the paradox of the 1990s [was] the apparent ubiquity of the rhetoric of radicalism at a time when the radical spirit seemed to have long evaporated' (Langan 1998: 214). For example, the concept of anti-oppressive practice comes from Radical social work and is now dominant throughout social work as a whole; yet the politicised structural understanding of power which Radical social work also argued for has largely disappeared. So, in this context, what does being 'anti-oppressive' actually mean? Has it come to mean simply being 'nice' to people?

The New Right and social work 'scandals'

The arrival of the New Right in the US and UK represented the end of the political consensus around the welfare state, and in Britain Social Work was on the front line of this. John Clarke has argued that there were two key elements within the New Right; an anti-welfarist strand and an anti-statist strand. From the perspective of the anti-welfarist strand, welfare spending was attacked on the basis that it was unproductive – a drain on the 'real economy' – and undesirable, in the sense of that it produced 'welfare dependency'. For the anti-statist element within the New Right, the problem was excessive state involvement in what should rightly be the role of the free market, which seen as the most efficient mechanism for allocating resources, goods and services (Clarke *et al.* 2000: 2–3). In order to achieve this change the New Right mounted an ideological offensive on the legitimacy of the welfare state, and social work came to be one of the main foci of this. This was achieved through a series of scandals about social work practice in which it came to be presented either as an agency so preoccupied with abstract questions of fairness that it was incapable of acting on the basis of common sense, or as an agency which, rather than helping solve people's difficulties, actually 'created' the problems it claimed it was solving. The scandals themselves all involved issues of child care and child abuse. As Rojek *et al.* noted in 1988:

> Nowhere have these panics been more severe, and more unremitting, than in cases of child abuse. For example late in 1985 the Blom-Cooper report on the death of 2-year-old Jasmine Beckford (victim of her stepfather). It identified serious errors on the part of social workers handling the case. The report prompted a series of scathing attacks on social work in the press . . . [In 1987] the death of Kimberley Carlyle (at the hands of her stepfather) provoked a full scale moral panic against social work (1988: 150).

These words were written in 1988, but since then these have become an almost permanent feature of the landscape. On the face it, these represent criticisms of alleged bad practice within social work. However, as Rojek *et al.* have noted, in the period of the ascendancy of the New Right, these came to define social work in the light of a central theme within New Right philosophy; which was that health and social care professionals, of which social work was taken as the exemplar, had taken power away from individuals, thereby creating a class (or an 'underclass' as it came to known) of people who are incapable of doing anything other than seeking handouts. Indeed the extent to which these attacks on social workers had become a form of popular 'common sense' in Britain was revealed following the death of Baby P., a child under the care of Haringey Social Services in November 2008, when *The Sun* newspaper ran a petition calling for the sacking of the social workers involved in the case, which was signed by over 850,000 people. As Iain Ferguson and Michael Lavalette noted of this:

> Initially the events were framed in a familiar guise: that 'politically correct' social workers were a 'soft touch' for manipulative parents; that social workers and their way of working were, at best, problematic, at worst completely failing; that there was a need for more regulation and controls over what social workers do; that the solution was more managerialism and marketisation of social care services (2009: 5).

However, they also note that as time passed evidence emerged of the dramatic fall in the number of child deaths over recent decades, as well as of an 'under-resourced childcare system where budgetary constraints and market methods of care delivery had made child protection, and social work generally, more difficult' (2009: 5). The impact of these scandals, which continue to this day, have been to place social work in the UK on the defensive, with politicians and media commentators finding it easier to make cheaply populist statements scapegoating social work rather than thinking more seriously about the difficulties involved in actually doing this work. Butler and Drakeford's work (2003) has pointed to the way these scandals have re-constituted UK social work in the image of this defensiveness through a 'symbiotic relationship between scandals, Committee of Inquiry and public policy' (2003: 4). They argue that as a result of this the present direction of social work practice is largely determined by perceptions of its failures as they are constructed by Committees of Inquiry. We use the term 'perceptions' because the voice of front-line social workers has been largely absent from this litany of blaming, over-simplification and pathology.

Case study

What makes a 'scandal'?

Butler and Drakeford's work on social work and scandals (2003) is useful for getting us to think about what makes a scandal so significant, or so 'scandalous'. They make the important point that not all incidents of malpractice turn into scandals; in other words there are particular circumstances which facilitate the creation of a scandal, and the way another situation of malpractice will be regarded as simply unfortunate. Scandals are, in other words, 'social constructions'.

Let us consider for example a railway accident which took place at Potter's Bar in Hertfordshire, UK, in May 2002, and which is known as the Potter's Bar train crash. When Britain's railways ceased to be state-owned and were privatised in 1993, responsibility for the maintenance of track and signalling was contracted out to a large range of different organisations. Many different organisations, including rail unions, expressed grave concern about the quality and consistency of the work, which was now carried out by a range of different groups, some of whom lacked previous expertise in this area of work. On 10 May 2002 faulty points installation resulted in one of the carriages of a train heading through Potter's Bar station coming off the rails and flipping into the air. Six passengers died as a result of the accident, with a seventh pedestrian killed by falling masonry. The private contractor responsible for this work, Jarvis, had inspected the faulty points the previous day, following concerns expressed by train drivers over the previous week. When this malpractice was investigated by the Health and Safety Executive the actions of Jarvis were heavily criticised, both by the Health and Safety Executive and the British Transport Police. It is revealing to note that an incident of cost-cutting and incompetence, which caused the death of seven people, never became the kind of scandal which changed the terms of policy, or came to define rail privatisation. Indeed it is revealing to note that while the social workers and social work managers involved in child care deaths are unlikely to ever work in the field again, newspapers reported in March 2011 that the Rail Regulator had dropped all criminal proceedings against the firm (*Guardian* 2011).

Questions

1 What is it that makes something a "scandal"? Why is it that child deaths in social work are seen to define the profession as a whole, yet by contrast the cost-cutting by Jarvis, which resulted in the deaths of passengers, never became a "scandal" in the same way?

2 Think now about incidents of medical or police malpractice, which are as frequent and as significant in their impact. Do these define those professions in the same way as scandals have come to define social work? Why?

3 In June 2011 a BBC documentary exposed the severe abuse of people with learning disabilities at Winterbourne care home, near Bristol. The care home was owned by a private firm Castlebeck, which runs 56 different institutions in the UK. The pictures of people with learning disabilities being abused by staff whose job it supposedly was to care for them was extremely distressing, and the incident caused outrage when it received widespread publicity. However, in thinking about incidents like this, the focus is often on 'bad people' who do the abusing, rather than on the wider conditions which make abuse more likely. What do you think these wider conditions might be? Is one of these wider conditions the fact that these institutions are extremely profitable for the owners? Is this likely to become part of the scandal around abuse in care homes? Why?

Conclusion

This chapter has sought to consider some significant moments in the history of social work, looking initially at the Victorian charity and the Settlement Movement as two of the most important streams which lead to the formation of social work. We characterised the tensions between these two traditions as a something which was carried over into State social work, when it ceased to be a voluntary activity and became a recognised part of the welfare state after the Second World War in Britain. The bottom-up tradition of the Settlements was very similar in spirit to the Radical social work movement of the late 1970s, in the way social workers saw the individual problems of people they were working with not as caused by their inadequacy as people, but rather as manifestations of wider social issues, expressed at the individual level. The attack on the welfare state initiated by the Thatcher government similarly harked back to the language of the Victorian charitable organisations, particularly for the way they saw welfare as undermining the capacity of the working class and poor to be self-supporting. This same tendency to return to and sentimentalise the Victorian period is equally demonstrated by ideas of David Cameron, a more recent leader of the Conservative Party. Using an idea he called the 'Big Society' he argued that all social welfare should be provided by volunteers, with the state not needing to get involved at all in this area of provision. It is in this sense that we see the way in which 'the past, the present and the future are really one', in the Harriet Beecher Stowe quote we used at the beginning of the chapter.

We would also note the significance of Butler and Drakeford's argument that social work continues to be plagued by this issue of scandal precisely because of deep-seated divisions over the meaning of social work amongst the political establishment (2003: 5) and within society at large. This is particularly manifested when children in the care of Social Services are killed; the way this is seen to reflect some inherent weakness within social work as a profession, rather than the extremely difficult nature of the responsibilities which front-line social workers negotiate on a daily basis, not to mention the compound nature of the problems facing the poorest people in contemporary society. Where does this leave social work in the present situation? The argument throughout this book is that social work's role in 'mediating the social' is as necessary and important now as ever. Social work practice still contains enough possibilities for improving the lives of individuals and communities to be committed to, and the further chapters in this book will seek to set out ways in which the challenges facing the present generation of social work practitioners can be thought about and engaged with. However, it continues to be the case that social work is constrained by the present political social and economic environment, and in particular the way in which values of individual aspiration and entrepreneurial competitiveness have triumphed over collectivist and social justice-oriented approaches. In this sense, the argument which is central to this book, which is that social workers need to be 'consciously ethical', is more important than ever. In the next chapter of this book we expand this argument by looking at what ethics and ethical framework are and how they work in social work practice.

Summary

In this chapter we began by looking at different definitions of social work and considered how differently these definitions described social work. The point we are trying to bring out here is that social work is not just one thing, but is rather a term that covers many different ways of understanding and dealing with social problems.

We then looked at the period of the 1890s and looked at two different sorts of social work – the Charity Organisation Society and the Settlement Movement. We examined these as a way of demonstrating differing ways of dealing with social problems. While the COS was certainly concerned at the poverty and degradation of life among the working classes they did not question the dominant order, and saw the social work role in terms of encouraging individuals facing difficulties to change themselves so as to adapt and conform to the status quo – in particular to become self-supporting, which came to be seen as moral duty, failing to grasp the exploitative dimensions involved in both paid work and the structural nature of unemployment. We contrasted this with the Settlement Movement, which worked around practical problems from the perspective of working-class communities as they saw and experienced them. Rather than seeing the problems of poverty and destitution as problems of individual character, they promoted a concept of social work based on campaigning and advocacy alongside practical measures to improve the lives of people. We characterised these two approaches as 'the two souls of social work': one representing a vision of social work based on the reform of individual character and support for the 'deserving poor', and the other representing an attempt to understand the circumstances of communities which experience poverty as a whole, and working alongside those communities in a collaborative manner.

We then turned to the period of the 1970s and sought to understand the contrast between mainstream social work and Radical social work as a later incarnation of those same tensions. We concluded the chapter by examining some of the difficulties social work faces within the post-Thatcher assault on the welfare state, and the way values of individual aspiration and entrepreneurial competitiveness have triumphed over collectivist and social justice-oriented approaches. In the face of this we argued that the key theme of this book – which is that social workers need to be consciously ethical – is more important than ever.

Further reading

Payne, M. (2005) *The Origins of Social Work,* Palgrave Macmillan, Basingstoke, 2005. While there are many books on the history of social work, this is the most contemporary and comprehensive one.

Lavalette, M. and Ferguson, I. (2007) 'The Social Worker as Agitator: The Radical Kernel of British Social Work' in Ferguson, I. and Lavalette, M., *International Social Work and the Radical Tradition,* BASW, Birmingham. For a book which looks historically at the radical tradition in social work, this publication is the most interesting and recently written one. Most of the essays in this book are relevant to this topic. In terms of the contemporary challenges facing social work, the issues set out in another book by those same authors are excellent: Ferguson, I. and Lavalette, M. (2009) *Social Work After Baby P: Issues, Debates and Alternative Perspectives,* Liverpool Hope Press, Liverpool.

There is also the excellent work of Rogowski, S. (2010) *Social Work: The Rise and Fall of a Profession,* Policy Press, Bristol.

For another attempt to offer an alternative future to social work see: Cowden, S. and Singh, G. (2006) 'The "User" Friend, Foe or Fetish? A Critical Exploration of User Involvement in Health and Social Care'. *Critical Social Policy,* November.

In terms of social policy a text which deals with these problems, in particular the way social work has come to be defined by scandals, is Butler, I. and Drakeford, M. (2003) *Scandal, Social Policy and Social Welfare,* Policy Press, Bristol.

CHAPTER 2

Ethics and values in social work

Chapter outline

In this chapter we will:

- Explore basic definitions of social work ethics, and outline some of the ethical dilemmas and issues inherent to social work practice
- Discuss the notion of value and explore the values base for social work as a key element in defining its specificity
- Outline some of the current standards and guidelines which promote ethical practice in social work

Introduction

For decades, ethical issues have been a problem for many social workers. In the UK, a variety of strategies have been developed to address the issue of social work ethics. For example, in the 1980s, a government committee was created to define social workers'.roles and tasks (National Institute for Social Work 1982). A White Paper published in 1998 on the modernisation of social services in England recommended the establishment of a Care Council in each of the four countries, a governmental body to regulate the practice and conduct of social workers and social practitioners (Department of Health 1998). A code of ethics for social workers covering UK-wide has existed since 1975, and a code of practice for social care workers is now forming the basis for social work and social care ethics in social care agencies in England with similar documents in Wales, Scotland and Northern Ireland.

Furthermore, many agencies and organisations offering social care and social work services provide their employees with staff handbooks, internal codes of conduct and ethical guidelines for practice. However, Strom-Gottfried and D'Aprix (2006) have noted that the plethora of codes of ethics and codes of conduct have failed to address explicitly the issues faced by those regulated by them.

Despite all these resources, social care practitioners have difficulty resolving ethical issues in their work contexts, and their experience shows that many ethical dilemmas still occur (Rhodes 1986, Banks and Williams 2005, Banks

2006, Pullen-Sansfaçon 2011). Social work practice, therefore, continues to be ethically problematic.

In this chapter we will begin to examine basic concepts that underpin social work ethics. Specifically, we will be exploring the notions of 'ethics', 'standards' and 'codes', 'values' and 'ethical issues and dilemmas'. Of course, this chapter is only aimed at introducing these concepts and illustrating them by practice examples, and much of it will be covered in more depth in the rest of the book.

First, we will begin by defining what ethics is, and situating it within two broad perspectives, that is, *prescriptive ethics*, and *ethics as practical reasoning*. We will then pursue by exploring the notion of values and value base in social work before looking at ethical dilemmas and providing some practice examples.

What is 'ethics'?

For thousands of years, many thinkers have tried to understand the world around them and articulate theories to help people discriminate between what is good and what is bad. Because knowledge always continues to evolve, you will probably not be surprised to hear that there are many of these theories, or ethical perspectives. Even the term 'ethical perspectives' could be open for debate, but in this book we will talk about ethical perspectives when we refer to theories and approaches that help us make sense about ethical situations and ultimately make a decision about what is good and what is bad.

As in the fields of sociology or psychology, there are many perspectives in philosophy and ethics to help you interpret and understand problems and issues around you. Simply put, different ethical perspectives could make you perceive an action as desirable while another perspective on the same action might be seen as less desirable or even plainly wrong. Some other perspectives would not tell you about the good or the bad action but instead would give you clues as to what makes a good person. The study of ethics has therefore developed according to different tangents in a similar way to the development of sociology in relation to the influences of Marxism, structuralism, functionalism and so on. Each of these different ethical perspectives, as applied to the study of social work, has their strengths and weaknesses, and each one provides guidance in understanding what is good or bad through different lenses.

What is an ethical perspective?

An ethical perspective is a way of seeing, which informs you about what is constituted as good or bad.

> **Did you know?**
>
> *Principle-based ethics* includes ethical perspectives that use principles or rules that help define the right and wrong action, whereas *character and relationship-based ethics* does not rely on rules to follow but instead focuses on the sort of person you are or the relationship you have with others. Some of these ethical perspectives are covered in Chapters 6, 7 and 8.

The following chapters explore a number of critical and ethical perspectives that will help you grasp social work ethics more fully.

Banks (2006) discusses ethics under two broader ethical perspectives: 'principle-based ethics', which includes Kantian and Utilitarian theories, and 'character- and relationship-based ethics', which includes Virtue Ethics, feminist ethics and ethics of care. Similarly to Banks (2006), Clark (2006) explains that social work ethics is ruled by three families of ethical perspectives, duty-based (Kantian ethics), outcome-based (Utilitarian ethics) and Virtue Ethics. In fact, that there is no formal agreement as to how ethical perspectives can be classified in social work and in philosophy more broadly. These will be articulated in more detail later in the book.

Broadly speaking, the concept of ethics is defined as the study of morality, that is to say how people define what is right or wrong, good or bad (Banks 2006). Specifically, ethics tends to be understood in two different ways (Clark 2000):

- As a *prescription* that dictates how to behave in problematic situations, which we will label prescriptive ethics.

- As a *discipline* that examines the foundations and the arguments on which the requirements are defined, which we will label ethics as practical reason.

Ethics as a prescription

The prescriptive type of ethics is one that usually tells you what to do or not to do. This type of ethics is well illustrated within codes of conduct that often surround us at work. This sort of ethics is very important in society because it gives people guidelines about how to behave. For example, think of something social workers should *not* be doing: engaging in intimate relationships with service users. Prescriptive ethics is there to remind you about that and to make sure that it is clear that this sort of behaviour is inappropriate in the context of professional practice. Prescriptive ethics is therefore essential to the good working order of any professional group, and any given society.

Prescriptive ethics is therefore very important. In the UK, social work practice is very diverse and varied and the different tasks social workers have to undertake are often highly influenced by where the work takes place. For example, a social worker working in a hospital will have a very different job than a social worker working for a small charity organisation providing services to homeless people. In this context, how do we know that one action is ethical from another which is not? Prescriptive ethics can help in this sense because social work is so diverse that it can be difficult, at times, to know if the action you are about to undertake is ethical.

In England, two codes of conduct are available from the General Social Care Council: one for employers and one for employees. The code produced by the GSCC is country-specific for England but each of the four countries has produced a similar version. The code of conduct for employers aims to complement rather than replace existing agency policies with many social care service providers (GSCC 2002a). It is the GSCC and the social care agencies that are responsible for reinforcing social care practitioners' compliance with the codes (Strom-Gottfried and D'aprix 2006). Compliance is also ensured by the process of registration of all social care workers and practitioners and by close monitoring of social care practitioners' adherence to the GSCC's six headings, which are:

1 Protect the rights and promote the interest of service users and carers;
2 Strive to establish and maintain the trust and confidence of service users and carers;
3 Promote the independence of service users while protecting them from danger or harm;
4 Respect the rights of service users whilst seeking to ensure that their behaviour does not harm themselves or other people;
5 Uphold public trust and confidence in social care service;
6 Be accountable for the quality of their work and take responsibility for maintaining and improving their knowledge and skills (GSCC 2010).

Codes of ethics and codes of conduct are important because they provide guidance to social workers and contribute to maintain the ethical standards to practice, at the same time than serving other functions: protecting and reassuring the public, legitimising social work's claim to professional status and fostering the allegiance of members to the profession (Witkin 2000). Together, codes such as one of the four Care Council's Code of Practice or the Code of Ethics for social work produced by the British Association of Social Workers (UK-wide) make up part of what we call prescriptive ethics.

Reflection break

1 Looking at the GSCC six headings, do you feel they can be applied anywhere, regardless of the context of practice?
2 How possible and desirable is it, in your opinion, to develop a code accepted by all to guide the profession?

We feel it is important to stress that a code of ethics, or even a code of conduct, should only be used as a general guideline to help you solve an ethical dilemma, or to give you parameters about ethical standards to follow in social work. Because practice is so varied, unless the code is very broad and general, one code of ethics will not always answer the needs of social workers who are practicing according to different methods or approaches, let alone in different types of professional social care settings. For example, the notions of confidentiality in working individually with a service user who belongs to a Traveller's community must be dealt with very differently than working in groupwork with young offenders. Therefore, one code of practice or code of ethics will, with difficulty, meet the specific needs of every type of dilemma met in practice.

Another important difficulty with using codes of ethics and codes of conduct is that they do not always clearly give the answer to an ethical problem. For example, it is not unusual to see one article conflict with another principle on a different page. To illustrate this point, a social worker could find herself faced with a difficult situation where a service user wants to stay home after a second hospitalisation from a fall: she may find that it is very difficult indeed to protect the rights and promote the interest of service users (heading one of the GSCC code of practice) at the same time than promoting their independence while protecting them as far as possible from danger or harm (heading three of the GSCC code of practice). This sort of difficulty, which emerges from conflicting principles within the same code of practice, was highlighted by Proctor *et al.* (1993) in their research in the USA. Indeed, they found that 85 per cent of the conflicts mentioned by the social workers reflected a conflict among principles listed in the National Association of Social Workers code of ethics in the USA (in Harrington and Dolgoff 2008). You are probably starting to realise that while code of ethics are helpful and very important, they are not always straightforward to apply in practice situations and therefore cannot be used as the sole means to manage ethical difficulties. To summarise our discussion prescriptive ethics is very important because it provides standards for practice, but it cannot be used as a sole means to ensure ethical practice across the board.

Ethics as practical reasoning

While we agree that prescriptive ethics is important, Clark's second category of ethics, that is, a *discipline* that examines the foundations and the arguments on which the requirements are defined, is equally, if not more, important to integrate in social work practice. Indeed, we believe it is fundamental for social workers to take some time to examine the basis upon which the codes and other moral norms (which are often used as the basis for prescriptive ethics) have been developed. Social workers have to be aware that just because a norm is formally accepted by a given society, it is not necessarily ethical.

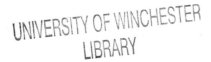

Many norms, whether formally or informally maintained in society, contribute to the *oppression* of some groups over others. Mullender and Ward (1991: 4) describe oppression as something that can be understood both as 'a state of affairs in which life chances are constructed, and as the process by which this state of affairs is created and maintained'. The term 'oppression' highlights an act of exploitation that can take a variety of forms (such as economic and social) and that has consequences that impact on the personal level for an individual but also on groups and communities. It is a process within groups that has power to limit, in an unjust way, the lives, experiences and opportunities of groups who have less power.

Oppression, although not necessary done on purpose, has an important role to play in the formation and the maintenance of norms in society. Therefore, even though prescriptive ethics is necessary and well intentioned, it has a trans-contextual quality that tends to favour people in socially advantageous positions. For example, many of the norms and rules that surround us contribute to reinforcing the social order and that social order is usually maintained to the advantage of the dominant groups, often consisting of heterosexual men, English-speaking, without physical or mental disability and belonging to a dominant social group, with good material resources and of Christian heritage (Sysneros *et al.* 2008, in Mullaly 2010: 198). However, it is by questioning and challenging these norms that we can contribute to developing a more ethical society according to a type of ethics based on practical reason. As Ricoeur (1985 in Bouquet 2004) suggests, there will be situations when struggles and value conflicts will evolve such that they eventually become recognised as new rights.

To illustrate this point, we could look at the situation of same-sex marriage in the UK. While not presently legal the UK, same-sex *marriage* continue to be the object of debates in public, religious and private spheres. However, it does not mean that because it is currently illegal the situation is necessarily ethical. Indeed, along with other forms of discrimination that many are still subjected to, gay, lesbian, bisexual, transgender and queer groups (LGBTQ groups) have engaged in struggles and legal battles to have their rights recognised legally and socially. In 1967 in the UK, homosexuality was legalised conditions of "consenting adults in private". This legislation has been subsequently built on in terms of legislation about rights to housing, inheritance, fostering and adoption, equalisation of the age of consent and in 2004 recognition of civil partnerships. This example shows how struggles and value conflicts can lead to the development of new rights that were previously nonexistent.

This argument takes us towards the need for a more reflexive type of ethics as described by Clark (2000), one that is based on the need to question the taken for granted ideas and the arguments on which the norm is defined. This is echoed by Clifford and Burke (2009) who assert that even though 'authority' establishes standards, principles and concepts, it does not mean that they must be accepted as ethical.

Codes of ethics and codes of conduct should be used as a reminder about the *values of the profession* but should never replace critical judgement. To be ethical in your practice, you will need to be critical in your reflexion while at the same time taking into account the legal, organisational and professional context in which an action takes place. In this book, we promote an approach to ethics that not only takes into consideration the professional norms and standards in social work, but also places practical reasoning in the process of ethical deliberation centrally.

What is a 'value'?

Looking at the literature on values, we note that the term itself is contested and that it is difficult to find one single definition. For example, a 'value' could be understood as a monetary concept rather than a unit to measure the content of a glass of water. In the realm of social sciences, *The Oxford Dictionary of Sociology* (1998) explains that values are related to ethics and ethical behaviour in so far as they connote ideas that people have about 'ethical behaviour or appropriate behaviour, what is right or wrong, desirable or despicable' (Marshall 1998: 689). Similarly, in social work literature, Clark (2000) explains that values are a belief that help people understand what is regarded as morally good and that are generally shared by different members of a community.

For the purpose of this book, we propose that a value is a strong belief that people adhere to. It is more than a mere opinion or preference and it can be personal, cultural, social, religious or organisational. A value may or may not be shared by all. Finally, a value can potentially influence a person's way of thinking and behaving.

As much as the concept of value is contested, exhaustive lists of values are also difficult to find. Indeed, many have proposed lists of key values which include differences and similarities between them. In fact, in doing some background research for this book, we found a website listing no less than 374 different values people may hold! While it is not our intention to produce an exhaustive list of values, we found that the work of Schwartz (1992) tends to be recognised by many as one of the most influential contemporary pieces of research of values: he effectively tested different sets of values among people from different nations, in their own languages. Although not all values were ranked

What is a value?

A value is a preference and a reference held by people about ethical or appropriate behaviour, about what is right or wrong, desirable or despicable and which governs personal and collective choices (Marshall 1998).

Table 2.1 Universal values and examples of related values

Universal values	Examples of related values
Achievement	Success, capability, intelligence, ambition
Benevolence	Honesty, forgiveness, friendship, meaning in life, loyalty, mature love, responsible, spiritual life
Conformity	Politeness, honouring parents, self-discipline, obedient
Hedonism	Pleasure, enjoying life
Power	Social power, authority, social recognition, wealth, leadership
Security	Health, national security, social order, reciprocation of favours, family security, sense of belonging
Self-direction	Freedom, self-respect, independence, self-determination, creativity
Stimulation	Excitement, novelty
Tradition	Devotion, humility, moderation, detachment, respect for tradition
Universalism	Social justice, wisdom, protecting the environment, equality, unity with nature, world at peace, broad-minded, inner harmony

Source: Adapted from Schwartz (1992) and from Pakizeh *et al.* (2007) – non-exhaustive list

equally by all, Schwartz nevertheless managed to provide a list of those values that were apparent in people's life all around the world. After all, attempting to identify some values that are more important than others could also contribute to maintaining the social order we discussed above. See Table 2.1 for a list of values provided by Schwartz.

As you can see from this list, there are different kinds of values, and some of them probably mean more to you than some others. In fact, you may have realised that some values may conflict with some other values presented above. For example, the value of humility may not always be compatible with that of social power. It may be difficult to have a strong sense of humility and moderation while at the same time having a strong inclination for social power and social recognition. But do values really matter in a person's life? How does it affect someone on a day-to-day basis?

Case study

Gill and Amy's understanding of the concept 'helping others'

Let's take for example Gill and Amy, two year-one social work students. Gill grew up in a middle-class family in Bristol after being adopted only a few days of her birth. Her adoptive parents have told her, since she was little, that she can get anything she wants in life as long as she puts the effort in. Yet as she grew older, she is struck by the 'luck' she had and decided to pursue her college study in social work. On the other hand, Amy had a difficult childhood. She had grown up in a family of six but always felt as though she never fitted in. She was overweight and the victim of many cruel jokes from her brother and sisters. She started self-harming at 12 and after noticing the wound, Social Services got involved in her life. Amy was prescribed antidepressants at the age of 14 as well as receiving one-to-one sessions with the school counselor. At 23 Amy has now resolved some of the issues she faced and decided that she wants to pursue a career in social work. At the entry interview, both said that they wanted to undertake social work because they 'want to help people'. During a classroom exercise in a year-one course, Gill and Amy and four other students have to discuss what 'helping people' means for them. Gill explains that for her, it is about working with families so that they learn to do better for themselves, for example, by getting opportunities to go to college so that they can reintegrate the labour market, get a good job and pay for all the things they need. Amy, on the other hand, says when she wants to 'help people', she means that she wants to make the world a better place, especially for kids who do not fit in. She wants to change things around her so that the children who do not fit in get accepted and do not have to go through a similar ordeal to hers. After a lengthy discussion, all the classmates realise that they all came to social work for mostly different reasons, even if at first they all look as if they share the same aim.

Questions

1 Why do you think two people like Gill and Amy have such a different view of helping people?
2 What do you think is the role of values in their career choice and their interpretation of 'helping people'?

Because values are beliefs that affect people in the way they look around them and judge what is right from what is wrong, it is possible, in the situation of Gill and Amy, that their values have a profound effect on the way they understand a simple concept such as 'helping people'. For example, because of her life experience, Gill may adhere strongly to the value of 'achievement' and 'self-direction' while Amy seems more inclined towards values of 'universalism'. As we have shown in this example, values have many practice implications: the value you hold may quite possibly affect every way you think, act and respond to situations. In fact, when you intervene in the life of a person, it is hardly possible to act entirely in an 'objective' manner. Instead, many of the values will influence your choice and decisions. Referring to other authors, Pakizeh *et al.* (2007: 458) stress that 'all aspects of individuals' everyday lives are influenced by human values (e.g., freedom and equality). People rely on these values by using them implicitly or explicitly to determine their future directions and justify their past actions, compare themselves with others, praise or blame themselves and others, take certain actions over other people and influence them and rationalise their attitudes and behaviour "(Feather 1992, Rohan 2000, Rokeach 1973, Schwartz 1992 in Pakizeh, Gebaner, and Maio 2007: 458)". Values, which can be personal, professional, social or even philosophical, are influenced by a multitude of factors such as age, gender, class, political awareness or affiliation and experience (Moss 2007).

This is why we believe it is essential that you initially engage, and continue to do so throughout your entire career, in a process of reflection about how the values your carry with you, personal, cultural, social, professional or anything else, will influence your intervention with a person, a group or a community. This is part of the process of engaging in ethics as practical reasoning that we claim is so important to social work practice.

Social work values

Even though there is no list of universally accepted values, there is neverthe-less one document that could be closely related to values and is accepted by most people: the *United Nations Declaration of Human Rights* (1948). Indeed, while this document does not explicitly state a set of universal values, it im-plicitly highlights some universal values such as freedom, dignity, equality and rights, that are taken as the basis for articulating the principles that follow in the *Declaration*. This document is particularly important for social work, be-cause the profession is known to have a special commitment to human rights which are taken as the base for the social work international code of ethics:

> Social work grew out of humanitarian and democratic ideals, and its values are based on respect for the equality, worth, and dignity of all people. Since its beginnings over a century ago, social work practice has focused on meeting human needs and devel-oping human potential. Human rights and social justice serve as the motivation and justification for social work action. In solidarity with those who are disadvantaged, the profession strives to alleviate poverty and to liberate vulnerable and oppressed people in order to promote social inclusion. Social work values are embodied in the profession's national and international codes of ethics (IFSW 2005 in IFSW 2010).

The British Association of Social Work (BASW) defines five core values for social work, and the ethical principles found in their code of ethics are derived from these values (Strom-Gottfried and D'Aprix 2006). The values are those of human dignity and worth, social justice, competence, integrity and service to humanity. As we will see later in the book, these values will be explored in detail and understood through different ethical perspectives. However, we want to stress at this point that the BASW code of ethics aim to express the values and principles which are integral to social work, and to give

Reflection break

1 Is it always possible to act according to all the social work values at the same time?

2 Can a practice that focuses on one value rather than another be considered ethical?

3 What are the constraints/barriers to deployment of these values into practice?

guidance on ethical practice. The code is binding on all members, and the Association also hopes that it will commend itself to all social workers practising in the UK and to all employers of social workers (British Association of Social Workers 2002).

Despite the disagreement of various professional bodies, social work worldwide is based around two basic principles identified by Lynn (1999) as 'personal caring' and 'social justice' (in O'Brian 2003). On the other hand, Banks (2006: 44–6) explains that the literature around the principles and values of British social work all revolve around the concepts of 'respect for persons' and 'service users' 'self-determination', a 'commitment to the promotion of social justice', and the concept of 'professional integrity'. These three values will be further articulated later in the book.

In summary, we want to highlight that the values behind concepts such as of human rights and social justice are fundamental to the profession. More precisely, Banks (2006) notes that values in social work generally include 'respect for the person' and 'the principle of self-determination', 'commitment to promoting social justice' and 'professional integrity' (Banks 2006), which are all related to the IFSW 2005 statement of social work values described above. These values are also expressed as key principles by the BASW and are widely echoed by many other country-specific social work professional organisations such as the Canadian Association of Social Workers, the Australian Association of Social Workers and the National Association of Professional Social Workers in India. While the meanings of these concepts will be examined later in the

Reflection break

We have now outlined a list of universal values (Schwartz 1992) and have identified what we can assert to be the social work professional values. Compare social work professional values with the list of values defined by Schwartz.

1 Which one is compatible?

2 Are there any values which are not compatible with social work?

3 Looking back your personal values identified in the earlier Reflection break, are they all compatible with the value base for social work?

book, we want to stress at this point that together these three concepts form what we would broadly call the value base for social work, although would agree with Petrie (2009) that these values tend to be Westernised and therefore will require social workers to question them and engage in a process of practical reasoning while integrating them. This will be explored further in Chapters 6, 7 and 8 of the book but at this point, we would like to emphasise that social work's value base is very important to ethical practice in social work and is a distinctive feature of the profession.

Values and ethical dilemmas in practice

In social work practice, there may be situations where some of the values or principles you hold may be in conflict. For example, Beckett and Maynard (2005) explain that 'values in tension' happens when societal values, agency values, professional values or personal values conflict with one another, when one or more values from the same category get into conflict. For example, a social worker may have to make a decision between taking action in order to protect an older person from abuse (protection of vulnerable people, societal value) and letting the person decide what is best for herself (self-determination, a social work value which is also a societal value). Similarly, a social worker may have to decide whether she breaks confidentiality in a situation where a service user is illegally claiming benefits while working (respect for the person through notions of confidentiality versus social justice or 'fair' allocation of resources).

A number of authors have attempted to categorise the different dilemmas that may emerge in social work practice. For example, Bouquet (2004) explains that ethical issues usually either highlight:

- An opposition between the law and ethics: you may think about a situation in which the ethical way forward is not necessarily the legal one.
- Tension between strategies for action and the law: for example, in situations where a social worker may be deciding to undertake an action which may raise legal issues.

What is an ethical dilemma?

A situation that highlights a conflict between two different courses of action or ways forward to resolve a situation.

Ethical dilemmas often involve a conflict of values, for example, between resisting something to pursue the value of social justice and the need to conform to others. We then observe that both actions are possible, but that neither of them are fully satisfactory.

- Conflicting stakeholder interests: for example, in a situation where a service user and a carer, or an organisation and a social worker, both have wishes and needs which are incompatible.

- Between methodology and ethics: for example, in a situation when a social worker may undertake a particular piece of work to achieve change, but the means to achieve it may be questionable.

These categories are, we think, quite interesting and broad enough to make sense in different contexts, but we feel that many practice dilemmas could fall in one or another category at the same time. For example, a social worker who has a conflict between the law and ethics may also experience a tension between their strategy for action and the law, practice and ethics being in dissociable. Banks (2006) also proposes four broad categories of ethical issues social workers may be confronted with. Like those proposed by Bouquet (2004), we think that some dilemmas could also fall within multiple categories and therefore the categories are not mutually exclusive. However, we believe they illustrate well

Case study 1

Issue around individual right and welfare

Vicky is a 28-year-old single mother with three children: Kevin is 8, Matthew is 6 and Becky is 3. Vicky has been seeing a worker called Jo through her Local Authority for the past six months because of difficulties in her new single-parenting role. Vicky and Jo have established a trusting relationship and things have been improving a lot at home since the beginning of the intervention process. While on the way to a home visit to another service user, Jo remembers that Vicky has yet to sign a form that is needed to apply for additional benefit. Because Jo is in the vicinity, she decides to stop at Vicky's to get the form signed if she is available. This way, the request for additional benefit will be sped up. After ringing the doorbell twice, noone answers, but she can hear Matthew and Becky's voices from the inside. The door is locked. After talking to the children through the door, Jo realises that the two youngsters are locked inside the house on their own while Vicky is away somewhere else. After 30 minutes waiting outside the house, Vicky is still not back. The children cannot unlock the door.

Questions

1 Do you think this is an ethical dilemma? Explain your answer and identify the conflicting values or positions apparent in the situation.

2 What do you think Jo should do in this situation?

3 According to your personal values, what would you do being Jo?

4 According to the social work values, how do you think Jo should react to the situation?

5 Is the response based on your personal values the same as your answer based on professional values? How are they similar? How are they different?

the type of dilemmas social workers have to face in practice in the UK. The four case studies that follow are the different categories of issues articulated by Banks (2006) as well as examples of ethical dilemmas to illustrate them.

In Case study 1, the dilemma emerging could be interpreted as arising from an issue of individual rights and welfare. While Vicky is self-determining and has the right to decide what is best for herself, she also has a responsibility to care for her children. The values of self-determination and protection are central to this case study.

Case study 2

Issue around public welfare

John works in a deprived area of an estate in northern England. He is doing some groupwork with young offenders to discuss solutions to address the issues they face. The project is funded by a national non-governmental organisation. After several meetings and some in-depth reflection, the group defines the problem as coming from the lack of resources for young people in the estate and are now working on defining strategies to improve their lives. In the light of the new budget and to reflect changes of priorities coming from central government, John's employer has to make the difficult decision to reprioritise the funding to different projects and consequently allocate the remaining funding to a project focused on working with the under-fives. His employer wants John to coordinate this new project and bring to an end, as quickly as possible, his work with the young offenders. However, the group of young offenders gets upset about the situation and decide to act and by holding a demonstration in front of the organisation. John's line manager asks him to stop the young people 'causing such a lot of trouble'. John therefore tries to negotiate with the group but they really want their project to work and are ready to do more to get it. They also blame John for not supporting them.

Questions

1 Do you think this is an ethical dilemma? Explain your answer and identify the conflicting values or positions apparent in the situation.

2 What do you think John should do in this situation?

3 According to your personal values, what would you do if you were John?

4 According to the social work professional values, how do you think John should react to the situation?

5 Is the response based on your personal values the same as your answer based on professional values? How are they similar? How are they different?

The dilemma emerging in case study 2 has many dimensions; most of them could be interpreted as issues around public welfare. There is the reallocation of budget to a different group of service users, both at the level of central government and the NGO. This could raise important ethical issues as to why one group is considered as more important than another and what would be the consequences of allocating, or not allocating the budget differently. Another level of dilemma is John's decision on the future of the young offenders group. He would probably need to ask himself what his responsibilities are as a social worker, an employee but also a citizen in light of these difficult issues. Overall we feel that this dilemma is interesting because it illustrates well the different dimensions that can be present in ethical issues and ethical dilemmas around public welfare.

Case study 3

Issues around equality, difference and structural oppression

Louise works for an independent project funded by the Local Authority. Her role is to facilitate sessions for women around any gender issues. The group was set up two years ago and many women have been participating since then. However, the group is open to new membership. One week, a new member introduces herself to the group. Her name is Rachel. Members of the group have some odd reactions to Rachel but nevertheless welcome her to the group. Two weeks later, when the women discuss the importance of their identity to their feeling of womanhood, Rachel discloses that identity is very important to her because she feels much better since she has finished all the medical procedures related to gender change. Rachel then explains that she had been biologically a man until about two years ago. After a major depression and much one-to-one psychotherapy, she had an inner need to live as a women. Following this she began a long and difficult process of gender change that she finally completed two months ago. She explains that participating in this group is very important to her because she feels she can understand other's women experience and validate her own through discussion.

Following this meeting Louise gets several phone calls from five of seven members of the group saying that if Rachel carries on participating, they will leave the group. No other resources exist around the area in relation to gender issues.

Questions

1 Do you think this is an ethical dilemma? Explain your answer and identify the conflicting values or positions apparent in the situation.

2 What do you think Louise should do in this situation?

3 According to your personal values, what would you do if you were Louise?

4 According to social work professional values, how do you think Louise should react to the situation?

5 Is the response based on your personal values the same as your answer based on professional values? How are they similar? How are they different?

Case study 3 highlights some clear ethical issues about equality, difference and structural oppression. First, there are the members expressing their wishes to exclude Rachel from the group, which could be symptomatic of discrimination and more broadly oppression coming from the society who traditionally sees people belonging to one or another 'sex'. Indeed, transgender people are often confronted with discrimination and harassment. Kosciw, Diaz and Greytak (2007) assert that from their research in the USA, 85 per cent of 'trans' young people have experienced verbal abuse and harassment on the basis of their gender identity. Furthermore, we note in the literature the many negative consequences related to coming out as different from a women or a man (Mullaly 2010, Hicks 2008). Hence it is very likely that the reaction of a number

Case study 4

Issue around professional role, boundaries and relationships

Kate works in a high school in a western suburb of Cardiff. Her role is to work with young people enrolled at the school who experience a range of difficulties ranging from personal to family and relationship issues. The young people who see her normally do so on a voluntary basis. During a drop-in session, Jade comes to ask questions about relationships. She explains to Kate that she met a guy outside of school a few months ago and that she is very much in love with him because he makes her feel special. She had sexual relations with him for the first time three weeks ago. Since then, they have been hanging around together with all of his mates and since she never had many friends at school, she find this new life very exciting. She also says that he has bought her lots of expensive things, like trendy clothes and a very nice gold chain, and that he has even paid for her new hair extensions. However, she is worried about her relationship with him because last week he told her that he would like her to go out, just for one night, with one of his mates and act as though she was his girlfriend. He says that this would be a nice way of paying him back for some of the expensive things he bought her, and to prove that she really loves him. Jade feels a bit odd about the situation because she does not really want to do it, but at the same time she would like to make him happy. After discussing the situation at length, Kate suspects that Jade is being recruited into a street gang and that her boyfriend is in fact initiating her into prostitution. Kate explains to Jade that she does not have to do that and that her boyfriend, if he respects her, should not ask her to do that either. At the end of the discussion, Jade appears distressed and tells Kate not to tell anyone what she has just told her. She says that if her boyfriend learnt about that, she could be in big trouble with him and his friends. Jade is 16 years old.

Questions

1 Do you think this is an ethical dilemma? Explain your answer and identify the conflicting values or positions apparent in the situation.

2 What do you think Kate should do in this situation?

3 According to your personal values, what would you do if you were Kate?

4 According to social work professional values, how do you think Kate should react to the situation?

5 Is the response based on your personal values the same as your answer based on professional values? How are they similar? How are they different?

of group members are directly linked to oppression, and that this situation perpetuates oppression as experienced by Rachel. On the other hand, it is possible that some of the women who express their difficulties with Rachel taking part in the group are genuinely related to their own feeling of oppression and the fact that they live in a society where men continue to be in a relationship of power over women. In this case, it may be justified for some women to be feeling oppressed themselves and for them, including Rachel in the group equals to including an oppressor.

Case study 4 is one that can clearly relate to issues about professional roles, boundaries and relationship in social work. Indeed, the social worker is faced with a situation where she could wish to build a relationship with the young person in order to better support her in her situation, but at the same time being confronted with a level of risk that could influence her towards disclosing the information to other professionals. It would also be relevant to check if the social worker had explained the limits of confidentiality before listening to the young person's story.

As we can see from the four case studies presented above, ethical issues can be varied and range from situations that are common in social work practice, and ethical dilemmas that often emerge as a consequence of a confrontation between two opposing sets of values or positions.

Managing ethical dilemmas in practice

An understanding of decision making can sharpen our awareness and understanding of ethical issues and lead to improvements in practice (O'_____ 1999). A brief review of the literature reveals a number of elements that impҳ on decision making for social workers in practice. For example, Boland (2006) asserts that the internationalisation of social work values, educational background, experience, prior ethics, training and professional identification of social work values all affect the decision making of social workers confronted with an ethical dilemma. Furthermore, group and organisational factors must also be considered in regard to individual decision-making behaviour (Karacaer et al. 2009).

Having said that, the more one adheres to a set of social work values, the more solid a frame of reference one can draw from in making ethical decisions in practice (Doyle et al. 2009, Pullen-Sansfaçon 2011). Furthermore, organisational rules often have a role to play in the decision making of social workers (Pullen-Sansfaçon 2011). To this end, there seems to be a tendency on the part of practitioners to rely mostly on organisational rules rather than to deliberate systematically in order to make a decision (Boland 2006). Rhodes was already arguing, in 1986, that bureaucratic norms, when too strict, can decrease moral responsibility in decision making and discourage reflective practice, which in turn can have a negative impact on ethical decisions and, in a broader sense, on ethical conduct. It is therefore necessary to also question the 'prescriptive' side of intervention. Similarly, O'Brian (2003:391) adds that with the rapid change in British social work through the development of new policies, regulations and guidelines, as "professional judgment becomes circumscribed [...], the social worker's role is somewhat different than ones that are based on the two values of personal caring and social justice".

There are many different ways to manage an ethical dilemma. Reviewing the literature, we found that a number of authors encourage the use of codes or ethics and of guides and tools to systematically facilitate decision making. Others favour a more reflective approach or focus on the importance of developing practical reasoning. Overall, we found that there is no best way of resolving a dilemma and that several debates continue to emerge in the literature about the most effective model for ethical dilemma resolution. One thing is sure: it is important to clarify your own personal values because they have an important part to play in decision-making processes. Throughout the book, you will be exposed to the process of practical reasoning, as well as some more systematic ways of managing an ethical dilemma.

Summary

We have now examined some of the basic concepts that are fundamental to understanding what social work ethics is, and have situated the importance of values in the development of ethical practice in social work. Through looking at different case studies, we have also observed that ethical dilemmas are situations whereby two distinct and often incompatible positions or values enter into conflicts. Finally, we have introduced the concept of decision making in ethics, and have outlined both the elements that may influence the decision and some of the ways ethical dilemmas can be managed. We will now turn to the second part of the book, which examines in more depth the different values and concepts pertinent to ethical practice in social work.

Further reading

Clark, C. (2000) *Social Work Ethics: Politics, Principles and Practice,* Macmillan, Basingstoke. This book discusses ethics and social work from a moral and political stance. It provides an interesting framework to understanding ethics and values in social work.

Banks, S. (2006) *Ethics and Values in Social Work,* 3rd edn, Palgrave-Macmillan, Basingstoke. This book provides a comprehensive review of ethics and social work. The section on codes of ethics is particularly useful because it provides the opportunity to examine values and principles in a contextualised framework.

Based on a recent investigation, Banks provides a stimulating analysis of the codes of ethics from 31 different professional associations across the world, considering the extent of their consistency and applicability to practice.

Moss, B. (2007) *Values*. Russell House Publishing, Lyme Regis. This book provides an introductory overview of values in the 'people' professions. Bernard Moss attempts to examine value-based practice's relevance for a number of professional practices, such as social work, youth work, nursing and the police, identifying some of the theoretical foundations and exploring how they relate to practice issues, with a particular emphasis on anti-oppressive practice and interprofessional work.

Part 2

THE SOCIAL DIMENSIONS
OF SOCIAL WORK ETHICS

CHAPTER 3

Power in social work

Chapter outline

In this chapter we will:

- Consider some of the complexities in defining power in the context of social work
- Look at the historic emergence of different ways of thinking about what power is and what it means
- Look at the views of power as they were expressed in the European Enlightenment, the work of Karl Marx, political struggles for gender and racial equality and the work of Michel Foucault
- Apply these ideas to a social work case, considering the relationship between ethical practice and power in social work

Introduction

The first two chapters of this book discussed the evolution of social work, followed by an examination of some of the most significant frameworks for ethics and values in social work. One of the most important issues running throughout this material is a crucial issue within social work: the question of power. As Roger Smith notes in his 2008 book *Social Work and Power*:

> Social work is not just concerned with direct interactions between service users, practitioners and their agencies, but is closely implicated in the conflicts and inequalities that characterise the contexts of their interventions, including those that reflect the wider forms of oppression and discrimination (2008: 7).

It is this sense of the way social work is *implicated* in questions of power, at the many different levels in which power is expressed and manifest, that we want to explore in this chapter. By using the word 'implicated' we want to suggest something more than the idea that social workers exercise power or have it exercised over them; rather we want to point to the way it is both of these, and often at the same time. As Smith has noted:

> [Social workers] are at one and the same time, acutely aware of their own relative powerlessness in an organisational and structural sense, and yet concerned as to how to manage their own authority over service users (2008: 17).

Smith is pointing here to the *ambivalence* of social work's relationship to power, and we see this as crucial. Ambivalence refers to the feeling of being simultaneously pulled in opposing directions, and this was demonstrated in the ethical dilemmas discussed in the previous chapter, as well as being a feature of many social work interventions. In Chapter 1 we discussed the way social work arises historically as a response to the persistency of problems which are essentially about power and powerlessness in society. Social work in that sense can be seen to arise from the desire of particular people to act as a 'power for good', to be an individual who can, as is said, 'make a difference' to these problems. The vast majority of people who seek to train as social workers are seeking in some way to rehabilitate those individuals who have been trampled on in the rest of society's rush to obtain wealth, status and security. But how do social workers understand and work with the problems they are presented with? This process of delineating the service user's problem through 'expert knowledge' is central to social work's mission. But is this process of assessing service users an exercise of power in itself? And if so, is that power exercised towards benign ends, or towards ends associated with social control of service users? How much are social workers able to respond to what they think a service user needs, and how much are their interventions determined by the rules, regulations and procedures of the organisation they are working for?

These are key questions in this chapter, and in this book, as questions of power interact very closely with social work's ethical framework. This is not least because the actions taken, or in some instances not taken, by social workers can have far-reaching implications in the lives of service users and their families, for good or ill. Power and ethics can be thought of as inseparable twins in a constant process of interaction, as the tensions between social work's idealistic 'helping' mission, the process by which service user's 'problems' are conceptualised, and the organisational and political pressures to which individual social workers are subjected, are played out. Ethical practice within social work is thus always contextualised within power relations, and this chapter begins by looking at the question of how power is defined, then moving to a historical discussion which looks at where our present conceptions of power come from. The chapter concludes with a social work example in which we try to exemplify the different conceptions of power discussed.

What is 'power'?

In an interesting discussion on the question of social work and power, Arnon Bar-On argues that 'if social workers are to help their clients, then they must master the discourse of power and use it effectively' (2002: 998). This writer is suggesting that social work is somewhat hampered by its ambivalent relationship with power, and this comment is just one of many discussions of the significance of power in social work practice. But before we can think about

What is power?

Power is a word we use all the time, but the definition of it is not straightforward. The *Oxford English Dictionary*, for example, lists no less than 15 different senses in which the word can be used. The most commonly understood meaning of the power is *'the ability to control people or things'*, and this is one of the most widely used definitions. However, when moving into a deeper discussion of power, this definition is really just a starting point for a longer discussion.

whether or not we agree with this statement, we need to ask ourselves, what do we mean when we are talking about 'power'?

In an influential essay on power entitled *Power: A Radical View* (1974), the sociologist Steven Lukes noted that the difficulty of defining power is that it is 'ineradicably value-dependent' (1974: 26). In other words, what you think of it depends on where you stand in relation to it; for instance, for those who have it, it can denote freedom, legitimacy, choice, autonomy and other positive values, while for those who lack it, it is can be experienced as exclusion, rejection, oppression and marginalisation. In this sense it is hard to come up with a neutral definition of power. While recognising this, Lukes goes on to distinguish between three key forms of power – power as *persuasion*, power as *influence* and power as *coercion* – arguing that although these are all quite different phenomena, we use the same word to talk about all of them. If we were to situate this observation in a social work context we could note that there is a world of difference between persuading a highly stressed mother who feels she has to cope with everything herself to accept respite care for her learning disabled son. The use of *persuasive power* here is something that potentially enhances both mother and son's capacity for meaningful participation in the community. This is different from, say, requiring a pregnant mother-to-be who is heroin-dependant to undertake treatment for her drug abuse. In this instance of *power as influence*, it is the institutional power of social work which gives the influence its significance. And of course social workers also possess *coercive power*, expressed most definitively in the powers to remove children from their families into Local Authority care. These examples point to the diverse contexts in which power is exercised in social work, and Roger Smith echoes this observation when he notes that this often makes it difficult to 'identify consistent underlying precepts which guide interventions' (2008: 2). Part of this difficulty can be seen to lie in the fact that power has these different manifestations in social work. A key issue within this concerns the *authority* social workers possess – and this is an issue which cuts across the three manifestations of power which Steven Lukes talks about – whether one is talking about power as persuasion, influence or coercion, all are reliant on an underlying sense of authority. The German sociologist Max Weber was one of the first of many sociologists who have been interested in the many forms of professional power

Power as authority

Max Weber (1864–1920) was one of the first sociologists to argue that we need to understand the issue of power through its exercise in the form of *authority*. He set out three different forms of authority: traditional, charismatic and rational-legal (see Craib 1997: 133–41 for a longer discussion of this). Traditional authority is vested in an individual on the basis of tradition and custom; the British monarchy or the Roman Catholic Pope are good examples of this. Charismatic authority is also vested in an individual, but this is exercised by virtue of their personality; think of African-American leaders like Malcolm X or Martin Luther King, whose soaring oratory and incisive analysis inspired people to join the political movements they developed. However, the key form of authority held in modern societies is what Weber called 'rational-legal' authority. This form of authority is not the possession of an individual, but is invested in a person on the basis of their being the holder of a particular office. This is the form of authority which is exercised by social care and health professionals in modern societies, which was additionally maintained through specialist training (Weber 2005: 214). Rational-legal authority, backed up by social work's recognised specialist role, is manifest throughout almost all social work interventions.

in the specific context of modern societies. Weber was significant for the way he tried to understand the nature of power *as authority* in societies.

Understanding power historically – the Enlightenment and its critics

We have begun by setting out some of the complexities in defining power, which derive from the way the word can be used to describe many different things at the one time. A useful way of clarifying where these different forms of power come from is understanding something about the origins of the way we think about power. This takes us on a historical journey into understanding how and where modern forms of power have come from. Having a historical understanding of these issues is valuable because the operation of power, however much we talk about it abstractly, is always *situated* in relationships between people, and between people and institutions, within particular societies. These relationships and the way they have been understood has changed considerably over time across different historical periods.

Medieval power and the European Enlightenment

In medieval Europe, power was vested in the figure of the Sovereign, and the kings and queens and members of the nobility who ruled Europe believed completely genuinely that they occupied their place as part of a divinely or-dained social hierarchy. This is the archetypal example of what Max Weber called 'traditional authority'. In this period, deference to authority and to the power of tradition was synonymous with obedience to the will of God. Sociologist Barry Hindess has noted 'in this view we are all born subjects' (1996: 13); in other words rather than seeing ourselves as being born free, but then having power taken away from us in different ways as people in modern societies generally do, the starting point in the medieval world was that we were born into a particular role in society, and for better or worse, it was that role that defined how our life would be lived. In this sense, people saw themselves as 'subject' to power as a consequence of the circumstances of birth. The idea of someone's status in a social hierarchy changing – say a very clever or hard-working peasant working his way up to becoming a member of the nobility – would have been seen as outlandish to people in this period, as the social strata in which you were born was seen to define your place in life almost entirely.

It was during the period known as the Enlightenment, which began in France and Scotland during the 1700s, that these ideas about a fixed and divinely or-dained set of social relationships were fundamentally challenged. This change came from a new grouping of journalists, writers, philosophers and activists. One of their most influential spokespersons was Immanuel Kant (1724–1804), whose writings on moral philosophy have had a huge influence and whose main contribution and influence on social work ethics is discussed more fully in Chapter 6 of this book. Here we want to discuss him in the context of the sig-nificance of these new ideas of power which developed in the Enlightenment. In a famous essay written in 1784 called 'What is Enlightenment?', Kant argued that the Enlightenment represented 'man's [sic] emergence from his self-incurred immaturity' (in Porter 1990: 1). Kant's work shook the founda-tions of the contemporary intellectual world with its particular assumptions of faith, tradition and authority, as he set out an entirely new basis on which these should be established. He argued that people needed to stop passively following tradition and established authority, but instead needed to see their lives and the choices they made as things in which they should be actively involved. Central to this shift was the idea that human beings were defined by the *capacity to reason*. Kant's key arguments regarding the importance of reason emphasised that it was the ability to possess and exercise reason which gave human beings the capacity to exercise free will. This was a crucial issue for all of the Enlightenment philosophers, and the historian Roy Porter has character-ised them as a movement which was:

> aiming to put human intelligence to use as an engine for understanding human nature, for analysing man [sic] as a sociable being, and the natural environment in which he [sic] lived. Upon such understanding the foundations for a better world would be laid (1990: 3).

The advocates of the Enlightenment called themselves 'philosophers', but far from being locked in ivory towers as we often think of philosophers, they saw themselves as a kind of intellectual political activist. Denis Diderot (1713–1784), another of their leading members, defined the 'philosopher' as a person intent on 'trampling on prejudice, tradition, universal consent, authority, in a word, all that enslaves most minds' (Porter 1990: 3). In other words, while the Enlightenment philosophers were very concerned with ideas, they wanted not just to share these ideas, but to change the societies in which they lived for the better by implementing these ideas. Another book which had a huge impact within the Enlightenment period was Jean Jacques Rousseau's (1712–1778) book *The Social Contract*, which was published in 1762. This book opened with the now famous words: 'Man [sic] is born free, and everywhere he [sic] is in chains' ([1763] 1998: 5). This statement sums up the Enlightenment's challenge to the dominant ways people had understood authority, which was that it was simply a given, and that to question these was in some way sacrilegious. By emphasising the idea that every person had the potentiality to think and reason for themselves, and to act accordingly on the basis of that, Enlightenment philosophers laid the basis for our modern views of morality and ethics.

Rousseau went on to argue that because people had this capacity for reason, the state itself should be organised on the basis of this recognition. Thus, the Enlightenment set the stage for a radically different means of understanding the relationship between the individual and the state. In opposition to the absolute monarchy of France, where the king saw himself as being placed on the throne by God himself, Rousseau argued that the only form of legitimate state order was one which was directly elected and accountable to 'the general will' (Rousseau 1998); anything other than this represented a fraud by the powerful upon ordinary people. It was the combination of these radically

Reflection break

Do you see yourself as the 'subject' or 'object' of power?

1 Think about your own life, and some key decisions you have made up to this point. Do you feel as though those decisions were made by you, or do you feel they were made for you?

2 Do you think of yourself as someone who has had a degree of control over how you have lived your life, or do you see yourself as someone whose life has been governed by other people's expectations of you and your role? Are you happy with this?

3 The fact that most of us will relate to these kinds of questions is a testament to the ongoing influence of the Enlightenment and its emphasis on free will. What are some of the things that prevent people exercising free will?

democratic ideas and the yawning gap between the opulence of the lives lived by the aristocracy and the poverty of ordinary people which laid the basis for the French Revolution of 1789. In the course of this revolution the aristocratic order which had dominated France for centuries was overthrown, and this event sent shock waves across the world. The aristocratic families that had controlled the reins of political power in Europe for centuries were challenged by revolts and insurrections from the newly emerging social groupings, as the ideas of the Enlightenment began to change the way people thought about political participation and power. The ideals of the French Revolution went on to have a major impact on the American War of Independence (1775–1783), as well as lesser known historical events such as the anti-colonial rebellion in Ireland led by Robert Emmet (1803), and first successful slave revolt in Haiti, which began in 1791 (James 1963), in which slaves also claimed their right to be treated as free human beings.

Georg Hegel (1770–1831), a German philosopher highly influenced by the Enlightenment and the French Revolution, took this concept of the centrality of the active rational subject still further in a book called *The Philosophy of Right* (1821). Hegel argued that every person simply by virtue of their humanity inherently possessed 'Abstract rights' (Houlgate 2005: 186). This could be seen as the origin of our present concept of human rights. However, Hegel did not just want to philosophise about rights – he argued that these rights needed to be made a reality through being enshrined by that state in a written constitution, and one which specifically sought to balance between individual needs and desires and more universal needs. Political liberty was also a key theme for the influential English philosopher John Stuart Mill (1806–1873). In a famous essay entitled 'On liberty' he argued that 'the only purpose for which power can be rightfully exercised over any member of a civilised community, against his [sic] will, is to prevent harm to others' (1989). The work of John Stuart Mill and other related thinkers, known as Utilitarians, was another important development for ethics in social work, and this legacy is explored further in Chapter 7 of this book.

New understandings of power: Karl Marx

The political world of the period after the Enlightenment was a turbulent one in which aristocratic monarchies crumbled in the face of popular revolt and new ideas of democracy and popular participation came to the fore. It was a period in which, as Andrew Bowie has noted, 'the tensions inherent in modern philosophy . . . became increasingly manifest as concrete problems in the socio-political world' (Bowie 2003: 118). Nowhere was this concern about the nature of the relationship between the world of ideas and the world itself manifest more strongly than in the work of Karl Marx. Marx's philosophical manifesto could be seen to be expressed in the words of his famous 11th 'Thesis on Feuerbach': 'The philosophers have only *interpreted* the world in various ways; the point is to change it' (Marx 2004). In other words, the validity of philosophy was not just at the level of philosophy itself, but in the way these ideas moved off the pages of books in libraries and into the real world of people's lives. This expresses one of Marx's key ideas about the way ideas, what is called theory, are realised through informing action in the world. The term for this is 'praxis', which means the unity of theory and practice, and this term was one Marx revived from the Greek philosopher Aristotle.

Marx is important in any discussion of the history of the concept of power, because he was both a product of the Enlightenment and one of its major critics. His work is hugely influenced by the Enlightenment, but he also marks out a new understanding of power which went beyond the aspirations of the Enlightenment philosophers. The distinctiveness of Marx's views can be seen by comparing the way he looked at Christianity with the views of the main Enlightenment philosophers. Like all of the Enlightenment philosophers, Marx was strongly critical of the Church as an institution. However, while the Enlightenment philosophers tended to dismiss Christianity as an 'illusion' which would disappear once people become more 'enlightened', Marx argued that you could only understand the influence it had amongst ordinary people by grasping the sense in which it spoke to their actual situation:

> Religious suffering is at one time the expression of real suffering and a protest against real suffering. Religion is the sigh of an oppressed creature, the heart of a heartless world and the soul of soulless conditions. It is the opium of the people (1975: 244).

Marx's description of religion as the 'opium of the people' has often been misunderstood to mean that he was simply dismissive of religion. Rather, he saw it an analogous to an opiate, in that it dulled the pain and struggle of people's lives, making carrying on a little more bearable. While the Enlightenment philosophers believed their devastating critiques of religious ideas and clarion calls for free thinking would finish off the Church as a force in society, Marx argued that instead you need to look at the real conditions of people in society, and it was only in this way that you could understand the appeal of religion. He argued that 'the abolition of religion as the *illusory happiness* of the people is the demand for their *real* happiness' (1975: 244); in other words, the problem with religion was not simply that is was an illusion, but rather its illusions were the veiled expression of a truth about power and exploitation which was too awful to contemplate, but which at the same time needed to be contemplated if this suffering was ever to be alleviated or changed. An example like this demonstrates the way Marx built on the insights of the Enlightenment but by grounding these insights in relation to the lives of ordinary people, it came to offer a much more radical understanding of the way power operates.

Marx looked at the Enlightenment theme of free will in much the same way. While he was entirely in favour of free will, he insisted on the need to move beyond talking about freedom and equality in the abstract and consider at the real circumstances of ordinary people – how much free will was possessed by a homeless family or a factory worker working a 12-hour shift? Marx's importance here lies in the way his understanding of power drew on Enlightenment ideas and values but took them one step further, seeking to locate apparently abstract questions in the real world of power and inequality. It was this which led Marx to conclude that the freedom of the property-owning classes was actually that which guaranteed the unfreedom of the working class – the class with nothing to sell but its labour, hence the need for workers to collectively discover their power *as workers*, and remake society so it was organised in the interests of the majority of people. These insights have acted as a major inspiration for the development of socialist, communist and trade union movements, including the Settlement Movement and Radical social work, discussed in Chapter 1. Marx's major contribution to our understanding of power, and an aspect highly relevant for social work, is that it is always embodied *materially*, that is, it always exists in social relationships, in particular the relationships between classes.

Who is a 'rational subject'? Issues of gender and 'race'

The Enlightenment philosophers saw freedom and equality as natural rights, but as Marx pointed out, most workers were trapped within coercive economic relations which meant that those rights could only become a reality if workers challenged and resisted those relations. If we think about the Enlightenment in relation to gender and 'race', the same issue is present. The working-class, women and people from countries colonised by European powers have all had to fight bitter political struggles in order to gain even limited access to the Enlightenment ideals. Why was this? It has been argued that a key explanation for this lay in the way the concept of reason came to be interpreted. As noted earlier, Immanuel Kant characterised the European Enlightenment as part of the process of 'man [sic] coming to maturity'; maturity in this context meaning the ability to use 'reason'. As Ramazanoglu and Holland point out:

> The dominance of reason put the reasoning mind in a position of mastery. The 'knowing subject' – the conscious self who reasons – could master the 'object of its knowledge' – the matter to be known. The natural scientist, the man of culture, could unlock the secrets of nature in order to master her. One consequence of this logic was to conclude that the rational, civilized, cultured man, with his access to certainties, could master the savage, primitive or barbarian, who was subject only to passion or a childlike mind (2002: 28).

In this view, the civilised mind came to be associated with the male members of the European educated classes: uneducated workers, and native peoples in colonised countries were seen as 'uncivilised' or 'barbarian', lacking the intelligence or refinement to understand or use reason. Women too, with their 'emotionally driven' natures, were equally seen as incapable of exercising reason. Stefan Johnsson has similarly noted the paradox of the way Enlightenment ideas were claimed as universal, but that the expression of this universality historically:

> reflected the specific values and interests of those persons through whom it is articulated. With few exceptions universal subjectivity had been articulated by white men of upper class background, and the resulting body of thought had been shaped accordingly: a mixture of humanist ideals and patriarchal values, universalism and racism, knowledge and bourgeois ideology (2010: 116).

This tension between universal values and the lived experience of most women during the years of the Enlightenment is revealing in this respect. The lives of most women at this time were lives of unceasing labour, both within and without the home. The ideas of the Enlightenment did influence the educational opportunities available to women of the middle and upper classes; however, as Richard Hooker has noted, the serious disciplines of science and philosophy were seen as reserved for men. For women, education was about the developing the 'accomplishments'; which meant various skills that contributed 'to the moral development and the "display" quality of a wife: music, drawing, singing, painting, and so on' (Hooker 1996). The famous novel *Pride and Prejudice* (1813) by Jane Austen demonstrates these dynamics through the story's focus on what constitutes a 'good marriage' for women of the propertied classes. Hence, while the Enlightenment emphasis on education greatly increased the numbers of people who were learning the new sciences and philosophies, the presumption was that women were not able to cope with these more serious disciplines and that they were unsuited for life beyond the domestic sphere. While men could master their passions through the use of 'superior reason', women were by definition located with the world of emotion and it was 'dangerous' to allow them to move out of that. Educated women did, of course, challenge these ideas, and one of the most notable examples of this was Mary Wollstonecraft's feminist manifesto *A Vindication of the Rights of Woman*, published in 1792. This document, still relevant today, makes a passionate appeal for women to be given access to education in particular, in order to end their marginalisation within the domestic world. Feminism emerged as a political movement in the mid-1800s, and one of the milestones of this was the Women's Rights Convention held in Seneca Falls, New York, in 1848. One of the central demands of this movement was the right to vote, and the bitterness of the political battle over the extending voting rights to women indicated how powerful was the idea that women belonged in the domestic sphere, rather than the wider public sphere. New Zealand was the first country where women were granted the right to vote in 1893, and in the UK women's voting rights were not made equal to men's until 1928. One of the most powerful accounts of the oppression of women was a book by the French philosopher Simone De Beauvoir, called *The Second Sex*, and first published in 1949. Her central argument is expressed in the memorable phrase that 'One is not born, but rather becomes, a woman' (1972: 267), and she argued that this process of becoming involves the internalisation of the idea that she is an object, forever defined as the 'other' in relation to a male 'subject':

> Humanity is male and man defines woman not in herself but as relative to him; she is not regarded as an autonomous being . . . Man can think of himself without woman. She cannot think of herself without man . . . With man there is no break between public and private life: the more he confirms his grasp on the world in action and in work, the more virile he seems to be, human and vital values are combined in him. Whereas woman's independent successes are in contradiction with her femininity, since the true woman is required to make herself object, to be the Other (1972: 262).

This work became something of a manifesto for the second wave of feminist activism which developed from the late 1960s onwards, and even though women have gone on to gain considerable numbers of political rights in wake of this, assumptions that women remain responsible for children and for the home, the other to the male with his focus on the external world of work, remain strong, even though large numbers of women now are working as many hours as the men they are living with (Hochschild 1989). It is in this as well as many other ways that the question of gender remains central to discussions of power, and this is particularly the case in social work. A contemporary example of this will be looked at the end of this chapter.

As we noted earlier, the fact that the pinnacle of reason came to be seen as the white male from the bourgeois classes was also significant from the perspective of the politics of 'race', since colonised peoples were similarly defined by ideas of immaturity, superstition and backwardness. Writers such as Frantz Fanon (1925–1961) and Edward Said (1935–2003) have famously characterised the way in which colonised peoples were never seen to be incapable of representing themselves, but could only manage in the modern world by being spoken for and directed by whites. In his 1952 book *Black Skins, White Masks,* Fanon spoke of the way colonisation created a situation in which black people were socialised into deferring to an image of themselves as inherently inferior to the white coloniser, based on a process of only being able to look at themselves through the eyes of the coloniser:

> I came into the world imbued with the will to find a meaning in things . . . and then I found I was an object in the midst of other objects. Sealed into that crushing objecthood, I turned beseechingly to others. Their attention was a liberation, running over my body suddenly abraded into non-being . . . But just as I reached the other side I stumbled, and the movements, the attitudes, the glances of the other fixed me there, in the sense in which a chemical solution is fixed by a dye (Fanon 1967: 109).

Fanon, who trained as a psychologist in Martinique, was one of the first theorists to fully chronicle the devastating effect this internalised sense of inferiority had on a black person. His later book *The Wretched of the Earth* (1961) was based on his involvement in anti-colonial political movements in Algeria in the 1960s, and had a major influence on anti-colonial and anti-racist movements across the world. Edward Said has addressed similar issues in his 1978 book *Orientalism*, which is concerned with the way people from 'the East' come to be defined and categorised by 'the West' as fundamentally alien to the West. The knowledge produced about the Orient, which is what he called 'Orientalism' is thus a 'western style for dominating, restructuring and having authority over the Orient' (1978: 3). The key point to which Said drew attention was the fact that the context of the colonised subject coming be 'known' by the West is the context of colonisation, where the indigenous people of those countries were economically exploited – slavery being the most extreme version of this – and denied political rights and representation. While most former colonies now have their independence, it is a mistake to think that these ideas do not continue to frame and shape our understandings of these issues. The contemporary representation of Islam and Muslims following the 9/11 bombings in New York and the 'War on Terror', where Islam was seen to be that which threatened the basis of the 'democratic West', could be seen to demonstrate Said's arguments. Just as women were categorised as lacking the capacity to reason on the basis of their inherent emotionality, racist ideas originate in this process of classifying people from colonised countries as inherently different and inferior, in short denying their capacity to think for themselves and exercise moral agency.

In this sense, the Enlightenment offers us an extremely important and at the same time contradictory legacy. It was only after a series of long and bitter struggles by the working classes that they gained political rights. There were equally arduous and bloody struggles fought by colonised peoples before their demands for self-government and self-determination were accepted by European colonial powers. Women also had to engage in political struggles of a similar order to gain the right to vote, access to education, to equal pay and to be able to enter the professions. In each of these cases, the dominant image of the working classes and colonised peoples was as 'savage' and 'uncivilised', just as the image of women was split between 'angels of the hearth', an idealised version of domestic life, and as 'hysterically emotional'. This relates to the legacy of the Enlightenment in the sense that savagery and hysteria were characterised as the opposite of reason, and therefore used to justify the denial of political rights. Nonetheless, because of the underlying universality of Enlightenment ideals, those same arguments came to be used by anti-colonial and feminist movements, when they demanded recognition of their rights as people and to argue for an end to colonial and patriarchal rule on the basis that these forms of oppression were against the spirit of the Enlightenment. In Chapters 1 and 2 there were a number of exercises which considered the question of whether ethical issues were universal or particular. Stefan Johnsson is interesting for his suggestion that rather than being thought of polar opposites to each other, as either/or, we need to think of these two as having a more interactive or both/and relationship. He argues that

> If there is today a global canon of universalism, it consists of documentary traces of past struggles in which oppression was resisted in the name of universal values. Like all canons, that universalism is selective and easily turned into a new instrument of oppression. Inevitably, every coding of universality is a *particular* representation (2010: 118).

The point Johnsson is making here is that universalism is a double-edged sword, and the dangers of an uncritical use of this can result in a high-minded ideal being used to justify oppressive practices. Nonetheless, it would be equally wrong to throw the universalist baby out with the bathwater. Universality remains important, not least for social work, because it implies the idea that as humans, we have something in common. At the same time, we may need to accept that rather than being fixed permanently across time and space, the nature of this connectedness is something that is revealed to us as we learn and grow, and as political movements emerge which challenge the things we previously saw as taken for granted.

Michel Foucault's theories of power

It is implicit throughout our discussion so far that modern ideas about power, upon which a profession like social work is based, derive fundamentally from the European Enlightenment and its intellectual and political legacy. It is for this reason that we have devoted later chapters to looking at the work of Kant, the Utilitarians and others, precisely because whether we are aware of it or not, these ideas derive from the frameworks which were set out here. The dominant assumption in the West is that these ideas represent *progress*; and while few would now deny that colonised peoples and women were treated as inferior in the practice of the Enlightenment, it is also true to say that these same ideas can be and were used as the basis for anti-colonial political movements as well as in movements for gender equality.

The French philosopher Michel Foucault (1926–1984) is significant for the way he has pointed to some of the lesser known abuses of people's rights which were justified through the language of the Enlightenment. Foucault's first work of major significance was a historical examination of 'madness', *Madness and Civilisation*, which was published in English in 1967. In this book he looks at the way that in the period after the Enlightenment, a 'Great Confinement' of 'the mad' within large psychiatric institutions took place. The placing of people with psychiatric problems in hospitals where they were treated by doctors has generally been seen as a step towards a more rational and 'enlightened' society, even if it is now acknowledged that many abuses of power took place within those institutions. Foucault, however, challenged this assumption, and argued that the rationale to exclude and confine 'the mad' was not only extremely oppressive, but also grew out of the Enlightenment's focus on reason as that which defined our humanity. Because 'madness' represented the polar opposite of this, the mad, who had lost the capacity to reason, were seen as less than human. In that sense the degrading treatment they received was not accidental, but a structured aspect of the way in which their situation was conceptualised and understood.

Foucault's book came to be situated within a wider literature which developed in the 1960s and 1970s, from former doctors and former inmates of psychiatric hospitals, as well as other commentators, concerned with the dehumanising impact of the large psychiatric hospitals and the abuses of power that took place within them. The work of R. D. Laing and Irving Goffman's highly influential book *Asylums*, published in 1961, were amongst the most significant writings within this. While Foucault did broadly belong in this camp, his concern was not just with madness, but with the power which was involved in placing someone in the category of mad. In order to characterise this he used the phrase 'power-knowledge'.

In a later book on prisons, called *Discipline and Punish* (1977), Foucault argued that the mechanisms for control and surveillance which are used in institutions like prisons were not just incidental to our experience of power. The use of surveillance as a means of creating compliance in population groups usually began amongst marginalised groups who were not well regarded by the rest of the society, such as prisoners or people with psychiatric problems, but were then extended to more and more areas of social life and government. This form of power which he called 'disciplinary power' was, he argued, amongst the most important ways in which power manifested in contemporary societies. In a lecture in 1976, Foucault argued:

What is 'power-knowledge'

This is a complex idea which is more than just the idea that 'knowledge is power'. What Foucault is trying to suggest is that knowledge, rather than being neutral, has an intimate relationship with power, and in particular acquires its status of 'truth' as a consequence of its use *within* power relations. The relationship between power and knowledge is thus a reciprocal relationship, in which power makes use of knowledge, which in turn reinforces the status of this knowledge. To take the example of madness, the knowledge produced in disciplines like psychology and psychiatry, while being presented as objective knowledge, is a form of knowledge which develops within the power relations of hospital settings and is itself an exercise of power over the patients of those institutions.

The judicial systems have enabled sovereignty to be democratised through the constitution of a public right articulated upon collective sovereignty, while at the same time this sovereignty was fundamentally determined and grounded in mechanisms of disciplinary coercion (1977: 105).

In other words, disciplinary power, a power which creates conformity and compliance through surveillance, represents a kind of hidden accompaniment to the Enlightenment philosophy of rights and equality. This represents a significant development to our contemporary understanding of power and is linked to his other important insight, and one very relevant to social work; the idea that knowledge needs to be understood as *always implicated* in the exercise of power, hence his use of the phrase power-knowledge.

What follows this case study is an attempt to think through the question of how a social worker might work with and respond to this situation with particular reference to the uses of power.

Reflection break

Think about a social work case example from your experience.

1 To what extent was the social work intervention used defined by the exercise of power? What sort of power do you think was exercised here? In whose interests do you feel it was exercised?

2 Are social work professionals' knowledge neutral, or are they as Foucault is suggesting, ways of exercising power over service users?

So far this chapter has discussed the definition of power, the historic emergence of particular ideas about power and various theories of power. We have made reference to the relevance of these to social work, and now we want to develop this in the case study in the final section of this chapter.

Case study

Joanna and Hannah

Joanna is a 30-year-old woman who lives with her daughter Hannah, who is 14. Joanna was 16 at the time she became pregnant with Hannah and was going out with Hannah's father Tim. Though they had been going out for over a year, and she knew Tim and his family fairly well, Tim has never become involved with Hannah, despite numerous attempts by Joanna to facilitate this. After having Hannah, Joanna lived in her parent's flat, while she attempted to finish school. This ended up being too difficult for Joanna, and after some time she abandoned school and decided to prioritise looking after Hannah. When Hannah was old enough to go to school, Joanna found work in a local supermarket. Once she had her own income, Joanna moved out of her parents place and got her own accommodation, a flat on the estate not too far from where her parents live. Things were going well for Joanna and Hannah until Hannah went to secondary school. Hannah's local secondary school was the one attended by almost all of the young people on the estate, and concerned at the school's poor reputation, Joanna made efforts to get Hannah into another school. She was however unsuccessful in this respect and Hannah attended the local school. This initiated a series of tensions between Joanna, who was increasingly critical of the girls Hannah was associating with, and Hannah's loyalty to 'her mates'. Hannah's academic work began to go downhill and various teachers began to express concerns to Joanna about Hannah's behaviour. This resulted in the relationship deteriorating still further as tempestuous arguments became a regular occurrence. These reached a new low point when Hannah stopped attending school altogether, and began to spend nights away from her home without informing her mother where she was. Social workers became involved with Hannah when the school took steps to exclude her following her persistent truancy and a fight in which she beat another girl quite severely. Hannah was charged with related offences and sent to a Pupil Referral Unit. A social worker became involved with Hannah at the point at which she was refusing to attend the Pupil Referral Unit, claiming it was a 'waste of time' and full of students who were 'thick'. She was at this point associating with a man in his early 20s who the police believed was involved in drug dealing.

After becoming involved with this case, one of the first actions a social worker would be likely to undertake is a core assessment. The findings of this assessment would then be reported at a case conference called by the social worker. In terms of the question of power, these actions are a demonstration of the social worker's *authority* both in terms of the expertise involved in undertaking the assessment and through the capability to bring about such a gathering of professionals and relevant others, including Hannah's mother Joanna. In the course of the case conference called by the social worker, they set out the view that the relationship between Hannah and Joanna has broken down, and that Joanna is currently 'beyond parental control'. The social worker, therefore, proposes that Hannah be required to attend a Local Authority residential unit. In terms of this conclusion the power of the social worker's assessment is again an expression of authority, which comes from the specialist knowledge on which social work as a profession is based. Max Weber would characterise this use of power as rational-legal, which suggests the neutral nature of professional knowledge, but this idea could be seen to be questioned by Michel Foucault's approach. His understanding of power would characterise these forms of professional discourse as power-knowledge; meaning that they are forms of specialist knowledge which through becoming generally accepted amongst professionals represent a form of power which allows an individual social worker to designate particular courses of action through the use of a particular label or category. This view could be backed up through Joanna's experience, where she would be only too aware that the social worker's assessment is not simply one view, but a view that carries significant weight and the power to define what happens in the lives of herself and her daughter. It is also the case that however much the social worker may see themselves as using their professional authority to keep Hannah away from danger and from potentially entering the criminal justice system, it remains the case that this professional view of Hannah's situation is one which is recognised and backed up by the power of the legal system and the state. This illustrates the value of Foucault's perspective in the way he makes us think about the implicit power involved in things like designating a child as 'beyond parental control'.

At the same time, an overemphasis on the coercive power which social workers undoubtedly possess can also be debilitating in terms of the process of initiating positive change in the lives of service users, and Foucault is not much help to us here. Social workers may find themselves at times taking actions that they believe to be in a service user's long-term interests, even if service users such as Hannah and Joanna see the social worker's involvement in their lives as unwarranted interference. However, we look at this situation: there has been a breakdown in the relationship between Joanna and Hannah, and Hannah, for all her bravado, is a vulnerable young person who needs help. The success of that which is offered will, to a large extent, come down to the thought and energy that her social worker is prepared to put into dealing with this. For example, how much has the social worker taken into account Joanna's account of why the difficulties between her and Hannah emerged in the first place? How much does Joanna feel her concerns and views have been heard? These points are significant at a deeply practical level, as the way these things are done is likely to substantially determine the course of events in this case, but they also show how important it is for social work practitioners to understand conceptually how close the relationship between power and ethics actually is. In this sense, it is useful to grasp Lukes' argument about the need when thinking about power to be aware of the impact of different forms of power, being aware of the way these different conceptions of power come subtly into and out of play. As noted earlier in this chapter, social work as an ethical enterprise remains very *implicated* in the exercise of power, and this relates to a theme we have sought to bring out in this chapter as a whole, concerning the need to be critical about the way power is being exercised – by ourselves, by the agencies we work for and by other agencies in the field with whom we are working. While organisational rules and procedures are important, as the discussion in Chapter 2 demonstrated, there is a tendency amongst practitioners to rely too much on these, rather than on thinking through the issues ourselves; we believe this is something practitioners and managers need to be very aware of.

In concluding this chapter we want to add one final dimension to the discussion presented so far, and this concerns a dimension of power which is both conceptual and practical. In the earlier discussion of the Enlightenment we referred to the way in which, while liberating on the one hand, it also showed that through characterising particular groups as not capable of possessing reason, the Enlightenment legacy was able to be used to maintain the power of new dominant groups in society – this was the group which Marx called 'the bourgeoisie'. The work of Marx and Foucault illustrates in different ways that in spite of an official ideology of democracy and human rights, the material power of one class over another (in Marx's case) or powerful assumptions about who is capable of reason (in Foucault's case), mean that the reality for less powerful groups in society is that their voices are rarely heard. Sociologist Barry Hindess expresses this same point another way when he argues that when we think about power there is always a tendency to explain it as 'the generalised capacity to act'. He suggests we need to see power as involving 'not only a capacity but also a right to act, with both capacity and right being seen to rest on the consent of over whom the power is exercised' (1996:1). In other words, power is not just about the ability to impose one's will upon others, it is also about the way the imposed power is accepted, often unquestioningly. This is important in thinking about the ethical use of power in social work situations, since it requires us to ask ourselves not only whether an exercise of power will be accepted, but why it is that acceptance occurs or does not occur.

In the previous example, we might think about the approaches which will facilitate Joanna accepting or rejecting social work intervention, but at a deeper level we also need to think about the unstated assumptions on which social work interventions often focus. In this instance, this is on the actions and behaviour of a mother, who has done what she could to raise and care for her daughter in the context of inner city life with all the pressures of low-waged work, single parenthood and schools where the staff are often overwhelmed by the demands upon them. In this context, it is the mother who stays with the child, rather than the father who does not, who is the object of professional attention. This reflects an unstated assumption, powerful in almost all cultures, that it is a child's mother who remains primarily responsible for the child. It is interesting that these assumptions would be likely to be shared as much by service users as by professionals, and this reflects our point about power and consent often resting on assumptions that are rarely examined. This is a crucial point when it comes to thinking about the relationship of ethics and power in social work, because it involves social workers having the ability not just to think about the most overt exercises of power by themselves and other health and social care professionals, but also the unstated assumptions upon which power is exercised.

Reflection break

Concluding reflection

Go back to the social work case you discussed previously. Think about the interventions that were decided upon by yourselves and others.
    Try to delineate the unstated assumptions behind your interventions.

1 Why do you think these remained unstated?

2 What would have happened if these assumptions came out into the open?

Summary

In this chapter we began by looking at different definitions of power and the difficulty of defining something which has such a complex nature. We also noted that the term actually describes several different processes, all of which are in play within the context of social work. In terms of the relationship between power and ethics we noted that it is important to be alert to this.

We then moved into a discussion of the different ways of thinking about power that have emerged historically. We looked at how power relations were understood in Europe prior to this, with their particular assumptions about faith and authority. We also looked at challenges to this from the work of Karl Marx, and political struggles for worker's rights, as well as the political challenge posed by struggles for gender and racial equality. Finally, we looked the work of Michel Foucault and his questioning of contemporary ideas about power.

We concluded with a case study in which we considered the relationship between ethical practice and power in social work. We ended by noting that a crucial point when it comes to thinking about the relationship of ethics and power in social work involves social workers understanding the expression of power not just in terms of a 'generalised capacity to act' but also through the power of unstated assumptions, noting how important it is for ethical practice that we become aware of and 'name' the way power is wielded through these.

Further reading

A crucial starting point for thinking about some of the definitional issues around power that remains Lukes, S., *Power: A Radical View* (1974), Macmillan, London.

Roger Smith explores some of these issues from a social work perspective in his book *Social Work and Power* (2008), Palgrave Macmillan, Basingstoke.

For further discussion of the European Enlightenment Roy Porter's book, *The Enlightenment* (1990) Macmillan, Basingstoke, is a good start.

Books on Marx are almost too numerous to mention but one that is historically based and accessible for a general reader is Osborne, P. (2005), *How to Read Marx*, Granta Books, London. The book on Michel Foucault in the same series, *How to Read Foucault* by Oksala, J. (2007) Granta Books, London, is also a useful introduction.

Books on the sociology of gender and 'race' are also widely available but a good introduction to feminist sociological approaches is Delamont, S., *Feminist Sociology* (2003) Sage, London. One book cited in this chapter is Frantz Fanon's *Black Skin, White Masks* (1967) Pluto Press, London. Written some time ago, it remains one of the most powerful and passionate explorations of the impact of 'race'. Because Fanon was himself a psychiatrist, the book has great relevance for social work, particularly in the area of race and mental health.

CHAPTER 4

The idea of empowerment in social work

Chapter outline

In this chapter we will:

- Discuss the changing uses of the term 'empowerment' and its significance for social work
- Develop a critical perspective on the different ways the term is being used
- Consider the relationship between a particular view of empowerment and the influence of neo-liberalism on social policy and service provision
- Consider the way these different concepts of empowerment can be thought about in the context of social work cases

Empowerment – that most difficult and noble of aims.

Robert Pirsig (1999) *Zen and the Art of Motorcycle Maintenance*

What is empowerment?

We have already noted the IFSW definition of social work as a profession which 'promotes social change, problem solving in human relationships and the empowerment and liberation of people to enhance well-being' (IFSW 2001 in Horner 2003: 2). This statement positions the concept of empowerment, alongside others, as the *raison d'être* of contemporary social work. But what exactly do we mean when we talk about empowerment in this way? The opening sentences of the social work academic and writer Robert Adams book *Social Work and Empowerment* offer some clue to this when he writes that 'Empowerment is a transformational activity. Social workers need empowerment to render their practice transformational' (2003: 3). Empowerment is about transformation, but to what? While the numerous writings in books like this give us a powerful sense that 'empowerment' needs to be right at the centre of what social work is about, it is not always clear what this actually involves.

However, there is no doubt about the popularity of the term in social work literature and policy; indeed in his 2008 book *Empowerment, Participation and Social Work*, Robert Adams lists 24 recent social work texts which have sought to 'apply the notion of empowerment to contemporary human services' (2008: 6). Yet despite the apparent centrality of the concept of empowerment to contemporary social work, Adams also notes that before 1990 it was a term that was barely mentioned in social work textbooks. Why then has this term taken centre stage, not just in social work theory and practice, but in contemporary social policy and political rhetoric? What does our present preoccupation with empowerment tell us, not just about the way social work is being framed and understood, but also about what is happening in society that gives this term such significance and cachet?

When it comes to defining 'empowerment' there are immediately a number of difficulties that we encounter. One is that the term carries such an aura of self-evident 'goodness' and positivity about it, it is often hard to question its use. But once we look beyond the assumption that empowerment is by definition a 'good thing', what we find is that the term is used to mean very different things in different contexts. Ward and Mullender were amongst the first to note this when they argued in 1991 that:

> empowerment has become the current bandwagon term in social work and is being used to justify what are, in fact, varying ideological and political positions . . . Broadly, empowerment is associated at one end of a continuum with the New Right's welfare consumerism, and at the other with the user movement which demands a voice in controlling standards and services themselves. One is the 'essential expression of individualism', the other rests on a collective voicing of universal need (Mullender and Ward 1991a: 21).

Mullender and Ward's argument is that the term is confusing, because it is being used to mean different things within different political rhetorics: it is about an idea of individual 'consumer choice' within the social welfare discourse of the New Right, but in the context of grass roots service-user movements, it is about disempowered groups having a voice. Alison Zippay, writing in a US context, has made the same observation. She notes that while historically 'efforts to empower poor people have traditionally been associated with liberal reformers . . . in an ironic turn of events, conservative Republicans have been amongst the most vocal and enthusiastic proponents' of the concept of 'empowerment'. She notes that this apparent paradox makes sense once conservatives have repositioned themselves as 'advocates of minimal government intervention in social problem solving', as they have from the 1980s onwards, since this allows them to 'hail the encouragement of self-initiative and individual choice and applaud the concept of local autonomy' (1995: 263). In other words, ideas about self-help and community activism, while being historically associated with progressive and radical politics, have now been harnessed by the political right as part of an overall attempt to reduce the role of the state in areas of social provision. This idea that it should no longer be the responsibility of state to intervene in social problems, as noted in previous chapters, is a key idea which emerges from the Reagan/Thatcher period in the 1980s–1990s, which leads to the emergence of what is known as neo-liberalism, with its emphasis on the 'free market', the individual and consumer choice.

Zippay notes that in this context the concept of empowerment appeals to contemporary policy makers and politicians because to them it represents people 'taking responsibility for their own lives', instead of 'looking to the state' to resolve those issues. However, as Zippay has noted, this represents a major shift from the terms' historic roots where it referred to the idea of greater community participation to 'enhance the democratic process', and ideas about 'the empowerment of disenfranchised community residents as a radical force for the redistribution of resources' (1995: 264). These latter views are distinct from the individualised view of empowerment espoused by conservatives, in that radicals argue that there is always a social dimension to problems of disempowerment (such as poverty, unemployment or domestic violence), rather than simply bad luck or fecklessness. The radical view of empowerment is therefore also about making demands on the state, including demands for more democratic access to resources. Both of these arguments from Zippay and Mullender and Ward imply that the success of the term 'empowerment' is that it is able to appeal to a wide range of positions across the political spectrum – almost everyone is in favour of it – but in reality it is being used to mean entirely different things in practice; hence when it comes to looking at concrete strategies to implement empowerment, the consensus around what empowerment means breaks down.

A key example which was used in the UK and the USA was the sale of state or local government-owned housing stock to the residents of those estates. This was presented by conservatives in the UK and the USA as means towards making people more empowered. What this meant was that instead of being so-called passive recipients of state-owned and controlled services, the residents would now own them themselves, and therefore have a supposedly more direct interest in improving the quality of life in those areas, instead of 'looking to the government' to do this for them. However, this proposal for the sale of state-owned housing was opposed by those on the left for the reason that, while it may be beneficial for those who were able to purchase the properties, the long-term impact of this policy would be to remove a significant quantity of housing which had previously been available for people on low incomes from the wider housing stock, making the poorest people more vulnerable in the housing market and leading to a major increase in homelessness. This reveals the different ways in which the term empowerment was being used: in neo-liberal discourse, the market is presented as empowering, while for the left, the market is seen as causing disempowerment, since state authorities which once accepted responsibility for reducing homelessness no longer have the resources available to do this. There is indeed considerable evidence that the sale of formerly state-owned housing as it occurred in the UK in the 1980s had exactly this impact on the housing market, and that the sale of this property, as well as creating a new class of owner-occupiers, also created another group who were excluded from the housing market altogether, creating a long-term increase in homelessness (see e.g. Allen 2007).

If we stay with this concrete example for a moment we could ask what this means in terms of how we might define empowerment. Robert Adams defines empowerment as 'the means by which individuals, groups and/or communities become able to take control of their circumstances and achieve their own goals, thereby being able to work towards helping themselves and others to maximise the quality of their lives' (2003: 8). While this sounds on the face of it as a progressive and democratic definition, the problem is that it could be argued that the policy of selling off council houses is entirely consistent with this definition; in other words, those people who were fortunate enough to be able to have benefited from this initiative have been empowered. However, what falls out of view, if we look at the situation simply in terms of this definition, is the wider more general picture of housing and homelessness. This illustrates a point made by Mary Langan regarding the use of term 'empowerment' in UK social work, which is that it implies 'an individualistic conception of power, which, by reducing social relationships to the interpersonal, obscures the real power relations in society' (1998: 114). Adams defines empowerment as individuals, groups and communities taking action to improve the 'quality of their lives'. But to address Langan's point, one of the problems with this definition is that it directs our focus to the group which is the beneficiary of a particular area of state policy, and in doing so obscures the reason why this policy has been adopted by the state, not to mention the implications that this has for other groups. This raises an important question about the 'goodness' of empowerment: if it is defined in terms of the benefit to a particular group or community, what does it mean if their empowerment is secured in a way that is to the detriment of another group or community?

Think about the following case study and the ways in which it manifests empowerment. In doing this exercise, read only Part 1 first and consider the questions posed. Once you have done this, look at Part 2 and consider those questions.

Case study

Part 1: Jane's story

Jane lives with her family in a small village in a rural area south of Birmingham. She is informed by her local residents association that there is a likelihood of attempts to erect buildings for which the planning permission has not been granted on an area of Green Belt land near her house. She feels concerned about this and is determined to stop it, and hence gives her details to the association to inform her of any activities they are organising in opposition to this. One morning Jane is telephoned by activists from the residents association telling her that builders have arrived on the site and would she be willing to join people from the village who are organising a blockade of the site. Jane drops what she is doing and joins the resident's protest. When the builders show the demonstrators documentation that proves the organisation behind attempts to build on this land does actually own it, the leaders of the residents association respond by asserting that the owners do not have planning permission. Some of the builders turn back, but others try to continue working until residents block the access roads around the site, when the demonstrators are removed by police. The residents association vows that the fight against the builders and the group behind them will go on even if it means facing arrest by the police.

Questions

1 Does an incident like this demonstrate an empowered group of residents?

2 How is this empowerment being manifest?

3 What kind of motivation do you imagine these residents had in acting in the way they did?

Case study

Part 2: Anna's story

Anna is part of large family of gypsy Roma travellers. She was born in Yorkshire but for some time she and her extended family have been travelling in an area south of Birmingham. Anna has five children, all of school age. For some time she has been trying to get them into various schools, but this has been hampered by the lack of a permanent residence, and bullying at a number of schools at which her children have attended. One of her sons also has asthma which is at times severe, and Anna would like him to be able to see the same doctor over a period of time instead of always visiting different Accident and Emergency departments when he has a severe attack. A group of the men in her family have been trying to acquire some land as a solution to the problem of always getting moved on by the police and hostile residents. However, the problem is that whenever they buy land and seek planning permission for building they find this is always denied once it is clear that the owners of the land are gypsy travellers. In frustration the group of travellers has simply decided that if planning permission is denied, they will go ahead and build without it. Hence a piece of land is purchased outside a small village, and planning permission is sought. Not surprisingly this is rejected; however, the group goes ahead and engages a building company to begin work as planned. On the morning the builders are due to begin work the group's caravans are parked next to the site, but the builders are prevented from

▶

beginning work because they are stopped by local residents blockading the site, carrying banners saying 'Keep off our Green Belt' and 'Stop the Invasion'.

Questions

1 Has your understanding of the situation changed at all having read Anna's story?

2 What attitude might you take to the situation now?

3 Thinking about contexts like this, does it mean that there are good and bad uses of empowerment? If so, how might we make that distinction?

The empowered citizen/consumer

Both Mullender and Ward and Zippay have pointed to the significance of the 1980s as a period where the term 'empowerment' was mobilised with very different meanings within different political discourses. This can be linked to the insights of Gail Lewis, which were discussed in Chapter 1. She argues that the 1980s was a turbulent period in which the welfare state was being criticised both from below – from user groups, grass roots campaigns and social movements like feminism and anti-racism, and from above – from governments with a New Right agenda for reducing the role of the state in social provision (Lewis 1998). Both of these political groupings were talking about empowerment, but with very different meanings and implications. These issues were resolved through the dominance of the critique of welfare from above, and the subsequent election of New Labour in 1997 represented the retention and consolidation of this agenda concerning the reduction of the role of the state. This has created a situation where the term 'empowerment', while beginning its life amongst the advocates of political change who were on the radical left, has now become part of the rhetoric of governments and policy makers pursuing a neo-liberal direction.

What is neo-liberalism?

David Harvey, author of *A Brief History of Neo-liberalism* (2007) has argued that the underlying theoretical justification for neo-liberalism is based on the view that:

> individual liberty and freedom can best be protected and achieved by an institutional structure, made up of strong private property rights, free markets, and free trade: a world in which individual initiative can flourish. The implication of that is that the state should not be involved in the economy too much, but it should use its power to preserve private property rights and the institutions of the market and promote those on the global stage if necessary (Harvey 2009, paragraph 4).

While this is the theory behind neo-liberalism, Harvey argues that one of the reasons why these ideas attained such prominence was as a result of a concern amongst powerful elites regarding the declining profitability of the economy and the need to restore this. In order to do this, the key strategy used when New Right governments attained political power was to undermine and attack the welfare state and unionised employment. While in the post-war period political elites had been committed to the maintenance of full employment, in the neo-liberal period this was abandoned, and as a consequence large numbers of state-owned manufacturing industries were sold off and privatised. The neo-liberal economic strategies deployed in the UK and USA in the 1980s caused record levels of unemployment. While this was justified as an attempt to bring down inflation, Harvey argues that these were in reality attempts to reduce people's sense of entitlement and thereby 'discipline' the working class:

> massive unemployment of course was disempowering for workers and at the same time . . . there was quite a massive loss of industrial jobs, manufacturing jobs, in the early 1980s. And of course that means less union power. If you close down the shipyards and the steel industry lays off people, then you have fewer people in the unions. The loss of jobs in the unionized sector disempowered the unions at the same time unemployment was rising; unemployment disciplines the labour force to accept lower paying jobs if necessary (2010, paragraph 6).

Neo-liberalism is currently dominant not just in economic policy, but in politics as well. If you are interested in understanding more about this, a good place to start is David Harvey's book *A Brief History of Neo-Liberalism* (2007).

Gregory Albo has argued that one of the key impacts of neo-liberal economic policy is social polarisation. The wealthiest in society benefit from the fact that there are huge remunerations for particular kinds of work, while 'annual wage increases [for the majority of workers] are kept below the combined rates of inflation and productivity'. Large groups of workers face 'longer hours of work . . . and the growth of informal and precarious work'. The latter are one of the main causes of the poverty trap, where people remain on benefits because the work available to them is so poorly paid and so intermittent that is not worth undertaking. The division between the workless and working sections of the working class also undermines the political solidarity which previously allowed workers to improve their social and economic position in society. This is combined with 'sharp cuts in welfare [which] fall especially hard on women and migrants', the groups which are hardest hit when benefits are cut or reduced. Albo concludes that to maintain existing living standards increasing numbers of people resort to going into debt, and the combination of this with 'privatisation and user fees for public services extend people's dependence on the market in aspects of daily life' (Albo 1988: 359). Alongside living in an increasingly polarised and divided society, which itself reaffirms an individualist mentality, neo-liberalism causes widespread levels of social insecurity as the safety nets which have been fought for historically to defend people against the vagaries of the market are stripped away.

In the context of what we can refer to as neo-liberal social policy, the concept of empowerment has not only become central, but has been linked to ideas about citizenship; that is, in defining the roles and responsibilities of citizens. The emphasis on the market, consumer choice and reduced role for the state in social care provision are now presented as permanent features of the welfare landscape and essential to delivering what we are told is 'what the public wants'. John Clarke argues that this ideological reconstruction of welfare has in effect 'de-collectivised' service users from being seen as *citizens with entitlements*, as they were understood under the welfare state, to *individuals seeking choice* in service provision. In this context, empowerment has become part of the rhetoric of 'choice', and he notes the way that:

> The imagery of choice both condenses and articulates a variety of desires for public service change and improvement – not all of which are about individualised consumerism. But choice links them as though they could be met through the singular means of empowering citizen-consumers to make choices (2005: 450).

Clarke is making the point here that people's desire for good public services which genuinely respond to their needs has become reconstructed as simply about the need for choice in public services, and in this framework, to be empowered comes to be defined as the capacity to act effectively within a market of consumer choices. The ideal of the citizen has thus become one who seeks to be an 'independent agent, rather than a dependant subject' (2005: 450), who wants to 'decide for themselves' rather than expecting the government to provide for them. While this rhetoric of community empowerment sounds on the face of it progressive and democratic, the notion of the good citizenship on which it is based implies a norm in which experiences of dependence come to be viewed in highly negative terms. This ideal of the empowered citizen, as Cowden and Singh have noted, often bears little relationship to the actual circumstances in which people come into contact with social welfare services. Who is it who will:

> represent the interests of those significant proportions of the population that are denied the status of citizen, such as asylum seekers or individuals with severe mental health difficulties? [With the State] having conceptualised its role as the facilitator and empowerer of essentially privatised communities, what happens when people in those communities fail to demonstrate 'appropriate' understandings of their role? (2006: 13).

The point here is that this new conception of the empowered citizen makes particular assumptions about individual capacities, wants and needs which often act to obscure the reality of new forms of exclusion and social division which are taking root as a consequence of neo-liberalism. Clarke develops this point when he argues that within our current economic and political situation there are broadly three different categories of citizens, whom he characterises as follows:

1 The law-abiding and hard-working majority, who are named, incentivised and rewarded. They are offered forms of choice and 'voice', provided this choice is exercised 'responsibly'.

2 Those who would like to be in the above category but are struggling to manage this. For these people what the state offers is 'a hand-up, not a hand-out' – that is there are government-sponsored interventions which seek to address their attitudes, character and motivation in areas in which they are seen as lacking.

3 Finally, there are those who are perceived as actively refusing to enter the world of the hard-working and law-abiding. These people become 'objects of intensified surveillance, criminalisation and incarceration in the drive to extend civility, reduce anti-socialness and enhance community safety' (Clarke 2005: 457–8).

Clarke's work suggests that our contemporary world of social work and social care in a post-welfare state situation is one where the Victorian distinction between the deserving and undeserving poor has returned with a vengeance. His argument about the way different groups of citizens are classified and addressed differentially by the state is one that has also been discussed by the social policy analyst Bill Jordan. Jordan's work is distinctive for the way he has sought to understand the power and significance of ideas about deserving and undeserving within the history of social work and social welfare. He argues that under these conditions where the gains of the post-war welfare state have been so substantially eroded, a new version of what it means to be a good citizen has emerged accordingly:

> In relation to mainstream citizens, the government is trying to nurture and develop certain psychological characteristics – motivation, self-esteem, confidence, entrepreneurship and self-development . . . to promote a self-improving form of citizenship [which] works on each individual to get them to have the right attitudes toward themselves, and to make the most of every opportunity that comes their way . . . Self-improvement, through work and in our private lives, becomes a requirement of citizenship (Jordan 2004: 9).

Jordan notes that these expectations are manifest through things such as education, where we are expected to get the most for our children, through health services, where we are expected to do all we can to maximise our own and our families' physical and mental health, and as workers, where we are expected to make ourselves as employable and flexible as possible. Following Michel Foucault, whose work was discussed in the previous chapter, Jordan calls this new approach to citizenship a 'project of the self'. This means that a sense of duty to fulfil these obligations is instilled internally, thus creating a situation where people aspire to live their lives according to these principles. Barbara Cruikshank argues that this process has become a key aspect of our present mode of being governed, which now concerns:

> securing the voluntary compliance of citizens . . . Technologies of citizenship do not cancel out the autonomy and independence of citizens, but are modes of governance that work upon and through the capacities of citizens to act on their own. Technologies of citizenship are voluntary and coercive at the same time; the actions of citizens are regulated, but only after the capacity to act as a certain kind of citizen with certain aims is instilled (1999: 4).

The people in Clarke's first category above are people who are seen to be the 'right kind' of citizens, and hence are encouraged in this. This means that the people in the latter two categories come to be understood not as people suffering particular sorts of structural inequalities, but as problematic individuals who need to be 'motivated and instructed in how to get their projects of the self started' (2004: 9). This latter point has major significance for social work because it works almost entirely with those sections of the community seen as least capable of acting in accordance with these norms of citizenship. In this respect, Jordan notes that there is an irony about social work's current rhetoric about empowerment and inclusion, since:

> in local authorities and other statutory agencies it is charged with motivating and cajoling these service users toward projects of the autonomy and self-development, while controlling those deviant and self-destructive aspects of resistance strategies (crime, drugs, benefit fraud, self harm, mental illness) (2004: 10).

Is empowerment 'good for you'?

This interrogation of the term 'empowerment' leads us to another really crucial question – is it meant to be something that you do for yourself, out of your own choice, or it is something that is done to for you or because someone else has decided that it is in your best interests? In other words, has it come to be seen as such a good thing that if you don't have it, it needs not just to be offered to you, but even imposed on you? This situation may seem paradoxical, but it emerges out of the way in which 'being empowered' has come to be positioned as an imperative of good citizenship in the landscape of contemporary health and social welfare interventions. Karen Baistow has argued that in the current period:

> Taking control of one's life, or particular aspects of it, is not only seen as being intimately connected with the formation or reformation of the self as empowered, *it is increasingly becoming an ethical obligation of the new citizenry.* Not being in control of your everyday living arrangements, your time, your diet, your body, your health, your children, suggests there is something seriously wrong with your ethical constitution.

Empowerment is not only good for you, it seems to be becoming essential to leading a better life (1994: 37).

Baistow notes that this sense of empowerment as an ethical obligation changes the way it is seen from an idea of empowerment as something which is good when people choose it for themselves, to the idea that if you do not choose it, this is because there is something wrong with you – we all 'need to be' empowered, and indeed if you don't want to be, then there must be some kind of flaw in your attitude or personality. It follows from this that if you are unwilling to act in a more empowered manner by yourself, then you may need to be empowered by someone else:

> My current reading of empowerment discourses indicates that . . . empowerment is something that is done to you by others, or that you do to others who thus become empowered by your actions not their own. Those who do the empowering are increasingly likely to be health and welfare professionals: social workers, health visitors, nurses, community clinical psychologists, psychotherapists etc. and managers in a variety of organisational settings. Those to whom empowerment is done are most likely to be users/clients/patients or employees. These are candidates for empowerment because in professional estimations they need it doing to them (1994: 37).

In other words, those who experience poverty, depression, poor housing or dysfunctional relationships are now seen to have a primary responsibility *as individuals* to empower themselves and solve their own problems. If they are unable to do this, then they need to be empowered through professional interventions. And it is here that the shift in the definition of empowerment within the neo-liberal policy universe becomes clear: empowerment has come to be about creating an ideal of citizenship where the citizen is an 'independent agent, rather than a dependant subject' (Clarke 2005: 450). Yet there is at the same time something deeply paradoxical about the way that it is professional assessments which designate first who needs to be empowered as well as the means by which this is to be realised:

> far from being left roleless, or less powerful, by the process of user empowerment, professionals are increasingly being seen as central to it in a number of ways . . . [which] confirm the mutual dependence of the professional and empowerment; firstly [through] the detection of suitable candidates in need of empowerment and secondly, the empowerment of them (Baistow 1994: 39).

Baistow concludes her analysis by noting the 'confusing and confused irony' of the fact that 'deciding who is to be empowered' is itself one of the most significant 'signs of power' (1994: 41).

The new discourse of empowerment can, therefore, be thought of as one which adopts the mantle of being progressive and democratic, but which essentially makes sense in the context of the state seeking to divest itself of historic responsibilities for redressing social problems. It is in this context that empowerment comes to be seen as the solution to problems of poverty, addictions, crime, parenting issues etc. As previously noted, this way of thinking about empowerment implies a particular version of citizenship – that of the hard-working and law-abiding – which is seen as that which needs to be adopted, or at the very least aspired to, by people living in situations of relatively greater material deprivation. But what this ignores is the different realities people experience; not just at the level of income, but also experiences of education, the kinds of ways in which people encounter the power of the state and how they experience that. Hence professionally defined empowerment strategies, which Jordan entirely realistically characterises as 'motivating and cajoling' service users against their deviant and self-destructive behaviour (2004: 10), are often unsuccessful. This is because this individualised conception of empowerment fails to grasp the way those problems, while manifested at the individual level, are socially produced. In the lives of people for whom 'begging, borrowing and stealing' are strategies for survival, it is the grinding reality of poverty which defines assumptions about what is possible. And what is particularly insidious is the way that when those strategies are seen to fail, it comes to be seen that it is those people themselves who are the failures, rather than our understanding of the issues.

Case study

The Khan family

In the context of work in your Children and Families Team, you are referred the case of Mrs Khan. Mrs Khan is 38 years old and originally from Pakistan. She lives with her husband, aged 54, who was born in the UK. The couple are married and have five children, aged 1, 4, 5, 8 and 11.

Until two years ago the family were getting along reasonably; however, a number of simultaneous difficulties have caused considerable problems for them. Mr Khan has worked for the last 15 years as a forklift driver in a factory not too far from where they lived. Two years ago he sustained an injury to his hand and arm which means he is no longer able to drive a vehicle or carry out manual work involving the use of both hands, such as lifting. Though the injury was caused through an accident at work, he has been unsuccessful in obtaining compensation and has had to go onto Jobseekers Allowance (JSA). Though there have been some jobs he could have done, the money he could have obtained for this work was less than the benefits he currently has, and therefore he has not seen any point in accepting them. One of Mr Khan's brothers has a shop and has offered some work to him. This does not bring in much money, but because he does not declare these earnings, he is able to use this to supplement his JSA. Mr Khan is extremely frustrated by his difficulty in finding work and as a result of his boredom and discontent he has begun spending many of his evenings at a local club where cheap alcohol is on sale and where many of his friends go.

Mrs Khan speaks little English and since she came to the UK she has spent most of her life looking after her children. Her caring responsibilities have increased in the last year since her mother was diagnosed with Alzheimer's disease; something which has caused considerable distress to her and her family. Whenever her father needed help he would telephone Mrs Khan in a state of considerable alarm, and she would feel it was expected of her to drop what she was doing and immediately offer support to her mother. The Khan family came to attention of Social Services as neighbours noted that the oldest child, 11-year-old Harbinder, was regularly looking after the younger four children while Mrs Khan was round at her parents' house, dealing with her mother, and Mr Khan was either working at his brother's shop or out at the club with his friends.

Questions

1 You have been given the case of the Khan family to work with regarding concerns around neglect. When this piece of work is allocated to you as a social worker, your team leader informs you that a duty social worker who made an initial visit to the family describes Mrs Khan as 'very disempowered'. In terms of thinking about how you understand the issues here, how useful is empowerment as a way of understanding and working with the difficulties she faces?

2 Looking at the issues she faces and the resources available to her, would you say that the strategies she has adopted for dealing with the demands on her are a realistic response to the situation she finds herself in, or an expression of her disempowerment? Why?

Empowerment and power relations

While strategies based on this understanding of empowerment can sound attractive, we need to be aware of the dangers in seeing this simplistically as the panacea for social problems. First, it can easily slide into the blaming of those seen not to want to be empowered; that their rejection, either actively or passively of professional interventions, leads to the conclusion that there is nothing more that they are capable of. In this way, the individualised means of conceptualising the term can end up reconstructing the distinction between deserving and undeserving service users – this is empowerment as a discourse of regulation. Second, by focusing exclusively on individual behaviour, we fail to grasp the significance of the way individual difficulties are socially produced. Under conditions of neo-liberalism, as we have discussed in this chapter, the economy has changed such that a significant section of the population is either excluded altogether from the labour market or has only a tenuous relationship with the world of work – low wages, hugely reduced levels of job security. At the same time, these people's experience of seeking state benefits is that they are both inadequate and punitive – and it is through processes like this that classes of disempowered people are systemically created. In order to understand the problematic aspects in the behaviour of these people which bring them to the attention of professionals, we also need to be able to ask the more fundamental question about what it is that leads people to act in ways that are violent, destructive or anti-social. The social theorist Slavoj Žižek addresses these issues in an interesting way in his book *Violence* (2009). In his investigation of this as a social phenomena, he argues that while we focus primarily on what he calls immediate 'subjective' violence – the violence that has a clear and obvious perpetrator – what we fail to see is the 'objective' violence – the violence which is 'inherent to the "normal" state of things' – which forms the backdrop to the former, but is rendered invisible by its very 'normality' (2009: 1–2). The challenge is to be able to understand the relationship between the two, and this brings us back to this question about the 'two souls of social work' discussed in Chapter 1. Do we understand people's problems as caused by the way they have failed to adapt to the brave new world in which we live, or are we able to locate the immediate problems in the wider context of the impersonal systemic exclusion which defines so many lives? What do these different understandings mean in practice?

A key issue in all of this is putting a critical understanding of power back into the equation. In the previous chapter, we discussed the problem with seeing power only as a generalised capacity to act is that this takes our attention away from the underlying assumptions about who feels they are or are not *entitled* to act; as it is these which define the everyday and normal operations of power. The individualised empowerment discourse which we have been questioning in this chapter not only obscures these wider questions but also makes the mistake of understanding power as a possession, which can be passed from one person to another. We consider the idea that you can *make* someone empowered is confused. In this sense, it is crucial that we adopt a critical approach to the use of terms like empowerment, which cannot be properly understood without first thinking about power and the nature of disempowerment as they are experienced in people's lives.

Case study

The case of David Fairbairn

David is a young man of 15 years old who has been referred to you for a court report for his criminal behaviour. He is also likely to be excluded from school for repeated incident of violent behaviour. David is part of a gang of boys of his age, which has been involved in a number of robberies in Kebab shops in the area of Birmingham where he lives. It has also been alleged that David has used a knife to threaten other boys at school to obtain mobile phones and leather jackets. David is white, but all the other boys in the gang are from black African-Caribbean backgrounds, and this is something which is commented on in the case notes you read before meeting him.

When you meet David you are struck by how friendly and charming he is. With little encouragement from you, he recounts his activities with the gang with great pride, and you are intrigued by the way he tells you how he has rejected the idea that he as a white boy should not be associating with black gang members – he is proud to be allowed into that world. David boasts to you that there are many criminal activities he is involved in for which he has not been convicted – particularly, theft of car stereos. He tells you that he steals these only from particular kinds of 'posh cars' and says that the people who lose them will 'get the money on insurance anyway'. He claims that he can get into a car and get the stereo out in less than 30 seconds, faster than anyone else in his gang and has the nickname 'Lightning' in his gang for precisely that reason.

In attempting to write your court report, you feel a strange mixture of feelings towards David. On one hand, you are appalled by the violence involved in his gang's attacks on the kebab shops and other pupils; on the other, you cannot help but feel admiration for him. Further conversations reveal his family situation. He has no contact with his father, and his mother has raised him on her own. His mother is currently studying accountancy to try to improve her circumstances and spends much of the time studying, often leaving David and his sister to manage on their own with little food and money in their flat. You cannot help but note that she has more or less left him to care for his younger sister, aged 10, and you are impressed by how caring and protective he is towards her.

Questions

1 Discuss your overall response to this young man and his situation.

2 As social workers, encountering people like David we often feel trapped between an idea of 'individual responsibility' and an idea of seeing someone's behaviour relative to the world or circumstances they are in. What are the arguments in favour of the 'individual responsibility' argument versus the 'relative circumstances' approaches? Which of these approaches do you feel is the most sound 'ethically'?

3 Might there be another way of working with a young person like David? What might an 'empowering' intervention with him look like?

In this chapter, we have tried to point to the problematic nature of the way empowerment has come to be used in social work today, linking this to the rise of neo-liberal policy assumptions. If that use of the term did represent an appropriation of an earlier usage, this raises the question of whether the term can be reclaimed more in line with its original usage for social work today. We want to conclude this chapter by thinking about this issue specifically in relation to the case study above. One point noted earlier is the confusion involved in thinking of power as an object which can be passed from one person to another. We have argued that power is a relationship – and Patricia Hill Collins expresses this in an interesting way when she talks of power as 'an intangible entity that circulates within a particular matrix of power relations and to which individuals stand in varying relationships' (2000: 274). The operation and experience of power in service user's lives is often quite complex and it is important for social workers to be able to recognise this. In his book *Challenging Oppression: A Critical Social Work Approach* (2002), Bob Mullaly argues that 'although there may be distinct *categories* of oppression, there is no oppression that creates a distinct *group* of oppressed people who are unaffected, one way or another, by other forms of oppression' (2002: 151). Power and oppression are only rarely about groups of oppressors and groups of victims confronting each other – it is more useful to think about the way power circulates not just between individuals and groups, but also within a particular person; so an individual can be simultaneously an oppressor and a victim.

The second key point we would make is that though power circulates it is also located. What this means is that it is exercised as well as resisted in specific contexts – in families, workplaces, schools and social settings. Empowerment, therefore, needs to be about the way individuals and groups situate and re-situate themselves in relation to specific located power relations. As Collins notes: 'As people push against, step away from, and shift the terms of their involvement in power relations, the shape of those relations changes for everyone' (Collins 2000: 275). What is crucial about this conception of empowerment is that people's capacity for self-realisation does not exist in a vacuum, but needs to be articulated within the particular social relations and networks of relationships in which individuals find themselves. Empowerment in this sense is concerned with the challenge to those existing networks of power relations, and while that is its most positive aspect, it is also its most problematic. Empowerment involves challenging other people, and that can make it difficult, scary or extremely risky for many people.

The Brazilian educationalist Paulo Freire has offered some insightful ways of thinking about these issues in social work. Freire is one of the most influential educational thinkers of the late twentieth century, and he advocated a conception of education based on dialogue between student and teacher. He argued that this changed the dynamic of education, offering the potential for the oppressed to regain their humanity and overcome their condition of inferiority. His most famous work, *Pedagogy of the Oppressed* (1972), argues for a system of education that emphasises learning as a practice of freedom. Freire began this book by characterising the disempowerment many people experience as based in what he called a 'double consciousness', and this is expressed by the way people are:

> at the same time themselves and the oppressor whose image they have internalized. Accordingly, until they concretely 'discover' themselves and in turn to their own consciousness, they nearly always express fatalistic attitudes toward their situation (Freire 1972: 61).

Freire saw this 'fatalism' as a consequence of people having internalised the dominant logic, and because the dominant logic *dominates* people's thinking and their perception of what is possible, it is very difficult for change to occur unless people have some space where they can reflect critically on how things could be different. Without this space it is very difficult to even accept that there are other ways of doing and being. At the micro level, people become locked into the perceptions and expectations or other people, while at the macro level it is endlessly repeated that there is 'no alternative' to the rule of the market over all aspects of social and economic life. In such a context, it is really so surprising that people's responses reflect this fatalism towards their wider situation?

Freire went on to define empowerment as 'the deepening and widening of the horizon of democratic practice' (Freire 1990). We want to conclude this chapter by thinking about the implications of this understanding in relation to the case study above. A key implication of this 'deepening and widening' is the idea of social workers being able to see the humanity within a service user, even if this humanity is not reflected in all of their actions. David Fairbairn embodies the contradictions of an individual who on the one hand demonstrates considerable insight, understanding and empathy, but on the other hand, appears to be able to switch this off and engage in acts of random cruelty and violence. His current situation is that he is on the path towards a career in the criminal justice system, which will reinforce, at both a subjective and objective level, that he has nothing useful to contribute to society. He comes to us not out of choice, but out of a lack of alternatives. We would suggest that a starting point for work is recognition of the real relations of power which shape the relationship between ourselves as professionals and him as the service user. A key concept in Freire's definition above is the idea of 'democratic practice', implying not just recognition of his humanity, but also that he is a citizen with political rights and the capacity for meaningful participation. However, this latter point would be meaningless to him in the absence of a space in which he can develop a wider understanding of his situation. In this sense, he needs to be *politicised* – based on an awareness of both the way the cards are stacked against people like him, and of the destructive and abusive nature of his own criminal behaviour – as part of a process of developing moral agency. The role of the social worker could be to initiate a dialogue which is based on uncovering or 'naming' the operations of power in his life, including the social work role itself, and in doing so creating a space where he can think about the significance of the way he uses and abuses power himself.

One possible objection to this course of action might be that it is patronising to work with David in this way; he knows his world and how to survive in it, what do you know about that? In an attempt to develop Freire's insights on empowerment, McClaren and De Silva make the point that:

A major consideration for the development of contextual critical knowledge is affirming the experiences of [service users] to the extent that their voices are acknowledged as an important part of the dialogue; but affirming [these] voices does not necessarily mean that [social workers] should take the meaning that [service users] give to their experiences at face value, as if experience speaks romantically or even tragically for itself. The task of the critical educator is to provide the conditions for the individual to reflect upon and shape their own experiences and in certain instances transform those experiences in the interest of a larger project of social responsibility (McClaren and Da Silva 1993: 49).

This quote is important for the way it emphasises the importance of a critical understanding of power and disempowerment as the basis for thinking about empowerment. Social workers hold power over service users, yet that power can be used in positive ways. As practitioners, we may not understand everything about the worlds in which people like David live, but we may one of the things we may be able to offer is a way of thinking about the wider social political and economic relationships which frame the choices he has. The social theorist Cornell West argued the purpose of this critical perspective is that it creates a space which 'allows suffering to speak. That is, it creates a vision of the world that puts into the limelight the social misery that is usually hidden or concealed by the dominant viewpoint of society' (West 1999: 551). A dialogue between the social worker and David could begin to address the unhappiness in his situation, as well as an understanding of what being in his gang offers him in terms of a positive form of self-identity. At the same time, David's activities within the gang are based on treating his victims in a cruel and dehumanised way. It is this ethical contradiction that offers the social worker a way of talking about what is wrong with his gang activities which does not simply involve seeking to motivate and cajole David towards a more respectable existence, an existence he has rejected just as it has rejected him. This form of dialogic social work both respects and interpolates his capacity to make ethical choices, at the same time as developing his wider awareness of his own situation, and in that process creating the possibility of other ways of being. The course of action proposed above may not have a guaranteed out-come – what interventions in social work do? In this sense it involves a risk, but not just the risk that it may be unsuccessful. It also opens up the risk that the social worker's position becomes open to interrogation from the outside, from the service user. To take this risk requires us to have confidence not just in our skills and abilities, but in the authenticity of our own critical understanding, and it perhaps this which is the most important element in any discussion of empowerment.

Summary

In this chapter, we have sought to open up the ever-popular term 'empowerment' and begin to question the idea that this is inherently a good thing in social work practice. The starting point of this is developing an understanding of the way this term is used to mean very different things in different political contexts.

The key issue we explore in this is the idea that the term begins in life on the radical left, but now finds its dominant use on the neo-liberal right. In other words, it starts as a term which is concerned with marginalised social groups and communities fighting to improve their situation. However, with the dominance of neo-liberalism, it comes to be used to mean people being freed from control by the state. For neo-liberals the state is bad – it is the free market which will liberate us. Hence struggles which were about democratising state provision come to be rewritten as struggles against state provision in favour of private provision. Empowerment, in a neo-liberal ideological world-view, thus comes to be about accepting 'personal responsibility', and while this idea is appealing at one level, it obscures the impact of the social dimensions of power, based on class, gender, race and ability/disability.

As well as opening up these different views of empowerment, the chapter concludes by arguing that a crucial dimension of conscious ethical practice is to reclaim this term as a means of understanding the relationship between individual behaviour and social oppression.

Further reading

For a clear and accessible understanding of neo-liberalism the best book is Harvey, D. (2007) *A Brief History of Neo-Liberalism,* Oxford University Press, Oxford and London.

For a more specific discussion of the issues in social work, the following are excellent: Baistow, K. (1994) 'Liberation and Regulation? Some Paradoxes of 'Empowerment'. *Critical Social Policy* 14 (42); Jordan, B. (2004) 'Emancipatory Social Work? Opportunity or Oxymoron?' *British Journal of Social Work* 31 (4). Jordan's other books, such as *Social Work and the Third Way: Tough Love as Social Policy* (2000), Sage, London and *Why the Third Way Failed: Economics, Morality and the Origins of the 'Big Society'* (2010) Policy Press, Bristol, are also well worth reading.

CHAPTER 5

Bureaucracy and social work

Chapter outline

In this chapter we will:

- Consider the importance of bureaucracy in modern societies
- Discuss the ways different theorists have sought to understand the impact of bureaucracy on ethical practice in social work, looking at *pessimistic* and *optimistic* accounts of this
- Consider the rise of managerialism and its effect on social work practice in the context of the shift towards neo-liberal conceptions of service provision and the importance of professional discretion in decision making

> In a modern state, the actual ruler is necessarily and unavoidably the bureaucracy.
>
> Max Weber (in Parkin 2002: 87–8)

> The main concern of too many social work managers today is the control of budgets rather than the welfare of service users, while worker-client relationships are increasingly characterised by control and supervision rather than care.
>
> (Social Work Manifesto 2006)

Social workers: prisoners of bureaucracy?

In July 2010, the UK Office for Standards in Education, Children's Services and Skills (Ofsted) carried out their first ever survey of children and families social work, *Safeguarding and Looked After Children* (Ofsted 2010). One of the most significant findings of this report emerged when the social workers interviewed were asked whether they felt that had 'time to work as effectively as they would wish to with children and young people': 64 per cent of respondents said that they did not, with one respondent quoted as saying that

> Workloads, expectations and demands on social workers are unmanageable. The majority of us are working long hours to simply keep up. This issue of long hours is 'hidden' due to the expectations of management and the ethos of disciplinaries. We are frightened to say that we cannot manage our workloads (2010: 13).

On further questioning, of those 64 per cent who felt they were unable to work effectively as they wished to with their service users, the main reason given for this was the amount of bureaucratic administration they were required to carry out, either in the form of paperwork or recording information electronically (2010: 14). These findings were reported on the BBC news website with the heading 'Bureaucracy Hampers Social Workers Survey Says', and in doing so, came to form part of a wider discussion about the way many public sector workers, nurses, the police as well as many others, feel they are spending more time 'doing paperwork than doing the actual job'. This is not the first time these concerns have been expressed in research into social work practice. In 2007 an almost identical concern was expressed through a survey of social workers carried out by *Community Care* magazine. In a report entitled 'Bureaucracy: Social Workers Bogged Down by Paperwork', this survey found that 'three-quarters of social workers spend more than 40% of their time on administrative work, including more than one-third who spend more than 60% of their working lives on administration'. So is it the case that social workers now are trapped in a quagmire of bureaucracy – or have things always been this way to a greater or lesser degree? How much is this a new concern and how much have these issues always been a tension in social work? The author of the previous article, Lauren Revans, makes the point that social work has always entailed a significant degree of administration, and she cites studies of social work in the 1960s and 1970s which she says illustrated that social workers then spent only about one-fifth of their time doing direct work. Rather than seeing the problem as bureaucracy as such, she suggests that what has changed is the nature of social workers administrative activities, where social workers see these as solely related to demands from managers in the sense of being unrelated to what they see as their job – which is doing work on behalf of service users. She cites Ray Jones, former chair of the British Association of Social Workers (BASW) who says:

> It's not so much about spending time with clients – I don't think that has changed. What I do think has happened is that more non-client time has been distorted. More of it is now spent on bureaucracy than doing things on behalf of clients (Revans 2007).

These recent examples illustrate the vexed relationship between the 'helping people' and the 'bureaucracy' aspects of social work. While this is a tension that we suggest has been around as long as social work itself, the form which this tension is taking may be becoming more acute for very particular reasons. It is these issues which form the focus of this chapter on bureaucracy and social work. We begin this chapter by trying to define bureaucracy, and our starting point here is the sociological writings of Max Weber, discussed earlier in Chapter 3 on power. Weber's work remains a crucial landmark in thinking about the significance of bureaucracy in modern industrial capitalist societies and for this reason it is important to understand his contribution. After outlining his ideas we then turn to one of the key ambiguities in his arguments, which concerns the question of who the bureaucracy is responsible to. This is a question which impinges directly on social work, and in particular the issue, which has been discussed previously, of who social work is 'answerable' to, both in a practical organisational sense as well as ethically.

This leads us to the question of how much social workers are controlled by the bureaucracy, or how much space the professional role gives social workers to themselves define what their role and tasks actually are. We approach this by considering the arguments of two different schools of thought, which we broadly categorise as *pessimistic* and *optimistic*. First we consider the arguments put forward by Margaret Rhodes in her book *Ethical Dilemmas in Social Work Practice* (1991). We class these as *pessimistic* in the sense that she sees an inherent contradiction between the needs of the bureaucracy itself and the needs of those whom it is supposed to serve, which she argues are almost always resolved in favour of the former. For Rhodes, the demands of the bureaucracy are what undermines social work as an ethical enterprise. The other side of this story, what can be characterised as *optimistic* arguments, follow the work of Micheal Lipsky in his book *Street Level Bureaucracy: Dilemmas of the Individual in the Public Services* (1980). Lipsky's distinctive argument is that while policy makers and managers never stop seeking to define and control what front-line professionals actually do, the very nature of the front line role means that they can never fully achieve this. Lipsky can be characterised as an optimist in the sense he sees *discretion* as ever present in the work of front-line professionals, who are forever in the business of inventing, improvising and working in, through, around and even against the substantive policy objectives of those higher up in the bureaucratic food chain.

The next part of our discussion brings us right up to the present and concerns the issue of whether contemporary social work is now subject to new types of bureaucratic control. These have been characterised by John Clarke as 'managerialism' and concern 'the forms of organisational control and direction, and the relations between leaders, staff and customers involved in the production and delivery of welfare outcomes' (Clarke 2000: 1). Clarke links the rise of managerialism with the impact of neo-liberalism on state policy, and this continues the discussion of the significance of neo-liberalism's impact on social work from the previous chapter. We conclude by asking whether these new forms of bureaucratic control are a key issue in the often-voiced dissatisfaction and frustration by social workers about the way they feel recent changes are so detrimental to the job, as exemplified at the beginning of the chapter.

Defining bureaucracy

What is a bureaucracy? Sociologist Max Weber is hugely significant because he was one of the first social theorists to talk about why bureaucracy has become such a pervasive feature of modern society as well as to define its central operating principles. Writing at the end of the nineteenth and beginning of the twentieth centuries, Weber was seeking to understand the phenomenon of bureaucracy; what it was and why it was that it had become so important. His key argument was that the rise of the bureaucracy needed to be understood as a consequence of the rational, calculating spirit of capitalism, which was leading to the emergence of new kinds of social organisations which were called upon to deal efficiently and equitably with large numbers of people. In our previous reference to the work of Weber in Chapter 3, we talked about the way he characterised modern societies as based on what he called 'legal-rational domination'; a form of authority in which authority is not the possession of an individual, but is invested in a person through their being the holder of a particular office. Bureaucracy was for Weber the most typical organisational form to develop out of a society based on these legal–rational principles. This was because unlike traditional or charismatic power, where power was seen to reside in the person themselves, bureaucratic authority is vested not in the person but in *the rules*. Frank Parkin explains that for Weber:

> The hallmark of bureaucratic domination is its studied impartiality. Its officials act without prejudice or passion, applying the same rules to all irrespective of rank or condition. The bureaucrat moreover is not the ultimate fount of the rule. Unlike the traditional or charismatic leader, the official in the modern state are themselves a servant of a higher political authority – typically an elected government and its ministers (Parkin 2002: 88).

While the centrality of impartial rules was crucial to Weber's view of the bureaucracy, he also saw the role of the bureaucrat in a large organisation as

---

Weber on bureaucracy

Weber defined the features of the bureaucracy as follows:

1 That it was a continuous organisation bound by rules.

2 That each individual in the bureaucracy occupied a specified sphere of competence.

3 That the organisation of offices follows a principle of hierarchy.

4 That the conduct of an office is based on the acquisition of technical skills.

5 That in the rational type of organisation it is a matter of principle that the people who administer the bureaucracy must be separated from ownership of the means of production.

6 That the administrators of the bureaucracy cannot appropriate their official positions.

7 Administrative acts, decisions and rules are recorded in writing.

From Craib (1997: 139–40)

representing a particular way of working. In his 1914 work *Economy and Society*, he characterised this as follows:

> The individual bureaucrat cannot squirm out of the apparatus into which he [sic] has been harnessed . . . In the great majority of cases he [sic] is only a small cog in a ceaselessly moving mechanism which prescribes to him [sic] an essential fixed route of march. The individual bureaucrat is, above all, forged to the common interest of all the functionaries in the perpetuation of the apparatus and the persistence of its rationally exercised domination.
>
> The ruled, for their part, cannot dispense with or replace the bureaucratic apparatus once it exists, for it rests upon expert training, a functional specialisation of work, and an attitude set on habitual virtuosity in the mastery of a single yet methodologically integrated function. If the apparatus stops working, or if its work is interrupted by force, chaos results, which is difficult to master by improvised replacements from among the governed . . . Increasingly the material fate of the masses depends on the continuous and correct functioning of the ever more bureaucratic organisations of private capitalism, and the idea of eliminating them becomes more and more utopian (Weber 2005: 214–16).

The point Weber is making here is that as a hierarchically structured organisation, bureaucracies define not just the remit and activities, but also the thinking of those who work within them. It is important to note that Weber's aim in discussing bureaucracy here was neither to criticise them nor to object to their existence; rather his objective was to argue that given the development of large-scale societies which had to process huge numbers of individuals, alongside the demands for rationality and efficiency in these dealings, the development of the bureaucracy was inevitable. In the above quote, Weber also notes another key feature of the bureaucracy; that it is based on the acquisition of technical expertise, and social work is just one of many examples of this. Weber saw society's need for bureaucracy as linked to the way we come to be dependent on bureaucratic expertise. Indeed when people complain about 'bureaucracy' and 'red tape', often what they are complaining about is not bureaucracy as such, but about bureaucracies which do their jobs badly. This becomes hugely inconvenient because of the extent to which we rely on them, and in that sense, Weber argued that the technical mastery of the bureaucratic office was invaluable to the smooth running of society. As the quote above demonstrates, he thoroughly rejected the idea that a complex modern society could ever do without bureaucracy however frustrating we may find our dealings with them.

After setting out these arguments mid-way throughout his career, towards the end of his life Weber came to see the development of the bureaucracy in a less positive light. While he never shifted from his view that bureaucracies were an inevitable feature of modern societies, he used the memorable phrase 'the iron cage of bureaucracy' as a means of expressing his concern about the vast impersonality of the bureaucratic organisation. He was particularly

concerned with the way a mechanistic loyalty to rules and impersonal specialisation could act to stifle individual creativity, independence and initiative. He
was also concerned about the way bureaucracies had grown and argued that
bureaucracy was absorbing everything – religion, music, art, war, law, education and family life had all entered the 'iron cage'; though it must be noted
that Weber would be rolling in his grave if he were to see the extent of their
expansion throughout the twentieth and twenty-first century! However, his
image of the iron cage remains significant for the way it expresses a particular
view of the modern rational world, dominated by a ceaseless search for efficiency. Weber saw this as a world in which charm, wonder and awe had disappeared, and he concluded his work on bureaucracy by noting that:

> So much more terrible is the idea that the world should be filled with nothing but those
> cogs who cling to a little post and strive for a greater one. . . . The central and further
> question is not how we further and accelerate it but what we have to set against this
> machinery, in order to preserve a remnant of humanity from this parcelling-out of the
> soul, and from this exclusive rule of bureaucratic life-ideals (in Pampel: 111).

It should be apparent from this brief account of his ideas that Weber has
bequeathed us a somewhat ambiguous view of the bureaucracy. On one hand
he argued strongly that there is no alternative to bureaucratic forms of organisation in modern, complex, urbanised and economically advanced societies.
How would the state and government keep track of the multiple activities of
its citizens without some form of bureaucratic organisation? However, the
comments he made about the stifling impact these could have both on individuals and on society as a whole suggest that though they may be inevitable,
this did not make them a particularly positive feature of modern society.
Sociologist Bryan Turner has noted that another key ambivalence in Weber's
work concerns the legitimacy of the norms which being followed by those
bureaucracies. Turner argues that it is one thing for Weber to insist on the
inevitability of bureaucracy as a means by which modern societies need to be
organised, but it is another thing to say what the rationale of this bureaucracy
is or should be (1996: 358). This is a question with substantial implications for
social work, because social work agencies are bureaucracies with the capacity
to intervene powerfully in the lives of individuals and families. Think of the
process of removing a child from their neglectful parents: this is a rationale
which claims to be about rendering assistance to a vulnerable child, yet this
process may be, and often is, perceived in entirely opposite terms by those on
the receiving end. It is one thing to say that we as a society would like such a
bureaucracy to protect vulnerable children – it is another thing to say that we
are happy with the way this or that organisation is undertaking this. Hence the
question of how bureaucracies treat people is a crucial question when thinking
about social work as an ethically based activity. This leads us to the question of

how we make sense of and conceptualise the actual day-to-day operations of policy and procedures for social work in the context of bureaucratic organisations, and it is to these issues that we now turn.

Understanding life in the bureaucracy: pessimists and optimists

While most books on social work ethics contain extensive discussion of different ethical theories, there is by comparison much less discussion of what we could think of as the 'real world' of ethical decision making, which is invariably located in the context of the bureaucratic agencies within which most social workers are employed. Margaret Rhodes' book *Ethical Dilemmas in Social Work Practice* (1991) is significant for the way she offers an extremely forthright discussion of bureaucracy, which can be regarded as one of the most distinctive contributions to this debate within the social work literature. In the opening pages of her chapter on bureaucracy, Rhodes argues that in a world in which public bureaucracies increasingly shape social work practice 'individual workers often seem caught up by organisational forces beyond their control', finding their work 'determined more by institutional rules than by client needs'. She also argues that in spite of the attempts by well-meaning people to improve the functioning of bureaucracy, the front-line social worker 'must continue to make her decisions despite inadequate resources, case overloads, excessive paper work, and a labyrinth of rules, all of which contribute to a sense of helplessness and hopelessness' (1991: 133–4). While these sentiments are ones that many social workers would agree with, the key question for our purposes here is to ask why this is. According to Rhodes, the fundamental problem is that:

> bureaucracies, by virtue of the kind of decisions they promote, undermine our ordinary concepts of morality. In particular, *human service* organisations undermine our moral concepts, because of their contradictory nature; their *stated* goal is to help clients, yet their actual operation serves the interest of preserving the bureaucracy. When this conflict is not recognised, workers often function as if their day to day decisions do not have ethical dimensions (1991: 134).

Hence, for Rhodes, the key issue is that there is an inherent contradiction between the ethical impulse of the social work professional as an individual, and the demands of the bureaucracy upon that individual.

She returns to Weber as part of her discussion on the basis of bureaucracy, and while she deploys the same categories for describing the bureaucracy as he does, she fundamentally rejects the idea that his description of the bureaucracy could simply be an objective description. The very features which Weber sees as those which allow the bureaucracy to work effectively, Rhodes characterises as the key factors which *undermine ethical decision making* in social work. To take, for example, the question of impartial decision making. While Weber sees this as a central feature of bureaucracy, Rhodes argues that this brings about a 'double standard' in that rules allow people to be 'freed from the demands of their personal moralities'. Consider, for instance, a situation where a social worker may personally believe that a particular service user is in need of support, but is also aware that the agency's eligibility criteria specify this at a particular level which that service user does not meet. Because the rules predominate over personal morality, the social worker dealing with this situation will feel that it is morally legitimate not to offer any further service to that service user because they do not meet the criteria for this support. The social worker, Rhodes argues, is able to see this decision as morally legitimate because they:

> do not hold [themselves] *personally* responsible for the action, because the choice is made *impersonally* by the organisation. The result of this split between personal and organisational morality is that an employee can dismiss general ethical considerations from evaluation of job performance (1991: 137).

At the core of Rhodes' argument is a powerfully expressed view that bureaucracies *through being bureaucracies* undermine an ethically based approach, as they are inherently based on a split between personal moralities and the rules and procedures of the agency concerned.

Another feature of the bureaucracy outlined by Weber is the specialisation of particular roles. Rhodes also sees this as undermining an ethically based approach in social work because it allows workers to only see themselves as responsible for the one part of the process which is their particular role, and in doing so they fail to consider the impact of different interventions on service users overall: 'Workers and agencies may spend considerable energy denying responsibility for a case . . . with the result that no-one will take primary responsibility' (1991: 141). An example of this could be a person with learning disabilities and additional mental health issues for whom neither a social services mental health nor a learning disabilities team is willing to take responsibility. While some might argue that the way to deal with this is to generate guidelines which specify what those agencies should do to avoid this happening, Rhodes argues that this is to miss the point about the way these forms of behaviour are inherent in bureaucracy. She concludes her indictment of bureaucracy by stating that:

> It may be argued that the failings of human service organisations do not result from bureaucratic structure, but from inadequate resources combined with increased demand. Certainly in this decade of new cutbacks to social programmes and higher caseloads, characteristics like impersonality of work and objectification of the client are magnified. These bureaucratic features, however, characterise human services whatever the political climate and are basic to bureaucracies as they are currently structured (1991: 144).

It is on the basis of this account that we have classified Rhodes approach to the role of bureaucracy in social work as *pessimistic*. It is important to note, based on her concluding statement, that she is not just criticising particular procedures which may be seen as unfair or discriminatory, or particular organisations which may do their job badly or treat service users oppressively. Her account locates the problem as *inherent in bureaucracy itself*. There is no doubt that many of the examples Rhodes gives will resonate with social workers; but the question we need to think about here is whether these issues are inherent in bureaucracy itself, or are the consequences of bureaucracies which function badly or treat people badly because they are shaped by powerful forces external to the bureaucracy. We want now to examine Rhodes' central arguments that the core of what is wrong with bureaucracy is this split between personal morality and bureaucratic rules through a case study.

Case study

Patience's placement

Patience is a social work student who has been living in the UK for six years after arriving from Zimbabwe as an asylum seeker and having now obtained the right to remain in the UK. She worked as a teacher before leaving Zimbabwe, and was inspired to train as a social worker after being helped by social workers in an asylum team. Prior to coming on the social work course, she worked for several years in a residential home for older people; she has also been involved in assisting other Zimbabweans who had recently arrived in the UK with practical and emotional support issues in work that she organised through her church.

For her first social work placement she joins a fostering team, and while she is very happy to have this placement, she is deeply shocked to realise not just that the team she works with places children with gay or lesbian couples, but that she may be herself expected to work with these people. The situation becomes clear to her after she undertakes a visit to a gay male couple with her Practice Assessor, Neelam. The couple she meets, Don and Warren, have done some short-term fostering with the Local Authority, which has gone extremely well. They are now interested in being assessed as potential adoptive parents. For Patience the visit to their house was extremely challenging in itself, and while she feels nothing personally against Don and Warren, the visit has raised a series of issues she needs desperately to discuss with Neelam.

At their next supervision, Patience explains to Neelam that 'as a Christian' she feels it is 'morally wrong to place innocent children with a homosexual couple'. While she has nothing against the men personally, their practices are 'against God's laws'. Neelam responds by saying she can understand where Patience is coming from, but as a social worker in training, she needs to think about social

▶

work values in relation to her own personal values. Neelam, who is from a Hindu background herself, says she felt similarly to Patience when she first trained as a social worker, but has since worked with several gay and lesbian couples, and now has absolutely no concern about it and indeed has come to champion the rights of gay and lesbian foster carers and adoptees as part of a wider campaign on issues of justice with the Local Authority. She says she feels proud that the Local Authority, having previously changed many of their policies on areas of race, have also now acknowledged the rights of gay and lesbian couples, many of whom are amongst their team's best foster placements. She offers Patience social work literature which explains these issues in more detail, as well as giving her a copy of the Local Authority's policy guidelines for fostering and adoption, pointing out that it is Authority's policy to welcome foster carers and adoptees from all sections of the community.

Questions

1 In a case such as this, should personal morality be allowed to predominate over organisational objectives? Why?

2 Consider this case in the light of Margaret Rhodes argument that the problem with bureaucracy is that it undermines 'personal morality'. What does this case suggest about that view?

3 Finally, consider the following outcome from this situation: after thinking long and hard about all the issues involved in this situation, Patience decides that in order to be successful on the social work course, she needs to accept that she has to work within the Local Authority guidelines. However, she cannot but feel that her own personal values have been compromised, and she explains this to Neelam. This leaves Neelam with the dilemma of whether or not to pass the case which they previously visited to Patience, as she was hoping to do. What do you think Neelam should do here?

We noted earlier that a key assumption in Margaret Rhodes' argument about the relationship between social work and bureaucracy is that individual morality represents a form of morality superior to agency policy and procedure. While this may be true in many instances, it is not universally true. This assumption, which is central to Rhodes' arguments, has been explicitly challenged by the sociologist Paul Du Gay in his book *In Praise of Bureaucracy* (2000). Du Gay characterises the position taken up by Margaret Rhodes as expressive of:

a thoroughly romantic belief that the principle of a full and free exercise of personal capacities is akin to a moral absolute for human conduct . . . [Within such a view] the specialisations of function and conduct attendant upon bureaucratic organisation are represented as introducing a violent 'split' into individual subjective and social being. The instrumental 'spirit of bureaucracy' makes fragmented . . . that which should be organic and 'whole'. It is because bureaucracy fosters only rational and instrumental human faculties . . . that it must be seen as a fatally flawed vehicle for the realisation of a moral personality (2000: 3).

Du Gay is arguing here that it is simply romantic to propose that instead of a bureaucratic structure for social work, social workers should be able to allocate resources to all service users on the basis of what they as individuals feel is appropriate – how would such an organisation function? Du Gay is suggesting, following Weber, that one of the great advantages of regulation is that it ensures consistency, and without this we would lack criteria for establishing what we considered was fair towards service users. He is also questioning the assumption that it is inherently unethical to take a decision which deploys one set of values in one setting and to use another set of values in another. Rather than this being something of an absolute distinction between ethical versus unethical decision making, as Rhodes suggests, Du Gay is suggesting that it depends on the context.

In terms of our case study above, imagine that after some time that Patience came to accept that in terms of her role as a social worker, she did need to be able to consider the qualities of foster carers and adopters regardless of sexual orientation. While such a shift would involve something of a split between her role as a social worker and her life outside of social work, is it right to characterise this as being based on an abandonment of personal responsibility or a rejection of ethical practice within social work (which would be the implication of Rhodes' arguments)? Du Gay is suggesting that because we live in a world which has 'different socio-ethical comportments', meaning that different things are expected of us in different situations, recognition of this is not the same as a distinction between ethical and unethical behaviour. Neither can it be simply understood as a split between a concept of personal responsibility and an acceptance of purely technical rationality (Du Gay 2000: 3). In other words, he is saying that in a complex and diverse world, it is commonplace that we make ethical decisions using particular criteria in particular situations and these may be different from other criteria we may use in other situations, but that doing this does not necessarily make our decision making inherently unethical – again that would depend on the situation we were in.

Indeed, Du Gay takes this argument about bureaucracy and ethics one stage further, and suggests that rather than being dominated by a technical rationality and thereby devoid of ethics, bureaucracy needs to be understood as an *ethical domain in its own right*:

> The ethical attributes of the 'good' bureaucrat – adherence of sub- and superordination, commitment to the purposes of the office and so forth – do not represent an incompetent subtraction from a 'complete' or 'all-round' conception of personhood. Rather they should be represented as a positive moral and ethical achievement in their own right. They represent the product of particular ethical techniques and practices through which individuals develop the disposition and capacity to conduct themselves according to the ethos of the bureaucratic office (2000: 4).

To put this point into the context of our previous example, one of the most important things Patience needs to learn as a social work student is precisely the question of *how to operate* within the bureaucratic office environment – the things she needs to do immediately and the things she can leave to do later, the things which are irrelevant and the things which must be followed up and pursued, the people she needs to develop a relationship with in order to get a particular process happening, the distinction between those procedures which must be followed to the letter and those where there is a certain room to manoeuvre. Du Gay is arguing that it is entirely mistaken to see the acquisition of these skills as involving a diminution of our own personal moralities – instead he argues we need to see the acquisition of these as crucial 'moral and ethical achievements' which will allow Patience to achieve what she has come into social work to do – help people.

So far we have set out what we have called the *pessimistic* view of the bureaucracy through looking at the work of Margaret Rhodes and considering its critique in the work of Paul Du Gay. Now we want to look at what could be called the *optimistic* accounts of bureaucracy. As noted above, these accounts are optimistic not in the sense that they suggest that everything that happens within bureaucracies is good – it is rather that they suggest that people within bureaucracies cannot be thought of as simply controlled by those organisations – but that people often have a certain room to manoeuvre. The key work which looks at this is Michael Lipsky's book *Street Level Bureaucracy: Dilemmas of the Individual in Public Services* (1980). Lipsky's work grew out of research which he carried out with front-line public service employees in the US – people such as teachers, police officers, social workers and public lawyers, whose role is to 'grant access to government programmes and provide services within them' (1980: 3). It is through this research that he has developed a distinctive account of the role of practitioners within the bureaucracy. Rather than seeing, as Rhodes does, that public policy *determines* the role of front-line practitioners, Lipsky emphasises the element of active agency exercised by front-line practitioners, arguing that it is their actions which in essence *make* that policy. He characterises front-line professionals as 'street level bureaucrats', and argues that:

> Most citizens encounter government (if they encounter it at all) not through letters to [their political representatives] or by attendance at school board meetings, but through their teachers and their children's teachers and the policeman on the corner or in the patrol car (Lipsky 1980: 3).

In other words, we experience the state bureaucracy not through grand statements of purpose and intent, or through the vast amounts of policy documents published by government departments, but through particular kinds of everyday interactions we have with state employees – teachers, health workers, social workers and police. These people are significant for the way they form the interface between the public on one hand and politicians and policy makers on the other. The argument of his which is most suggestive in the context of our discussion here is the idea that each one of these everyday interactions between the public and front-line practitioners

> represents an instance of policy delivery . . . Although [front line practitioners] are normally regarded as low-level employees, the actions of most public service workers actually constitute the services 'delivered' by government. Moreover when taken to-gether the individual decisions of these workers become, or add up to, agency policy (1980: 3).

It follows from Lispsky's argument that one of the reasons why front-line professionals such as police, social workers, teachers and health professionals are so often controversial figures, frequently in the news and singled out for either criticism or praise by politicians and other commentators, is that the decisions they make, frequently in situations of considerable stress, can have a massive impact on the people on the receiving end. As Lipsky notes:

> in delivering policy, street level bureaucrats made decisions about people that affect their life chances. To designate or treat someone as a welfare recipient, a juvenile de-linquent, or a high achiever affects the relationships of others to that person and also affects the person's self evaluation . . . A defining feature of the working environment of street level bureaucrats is that they must deal with client's personal reactions to their decisions . . . [and this means that] the reality of the work of street level bureau-crats could hardly be farther from the bureaucratic ideal of impersonal detachment in decision making (1980: 9).

Lipsky is emphasising that rather than seeing street level bureaucrats as *defined* by the rules and procedures they work within, as both Weber and Margaret Rhodes argue, it makes more sense to see them as *intermediaries* between policy guidelines and the public. In the context of social work, one of the most significant skills the social worker has to acquire is how to carry out this mediating role between the wider bureaucracy, to which they are formally accountable, and to the service user, to whom they are also accountable. This accountability is both formal – in the sense that an agency employs a social worker and could terminate this employment if the employee's behaviour was seen to be inappropriate – and ethical in that the social worker is likely to feel a sense of responsibility to both the from agency and to the service user. How the social worker and their agency experience this sense of duty may vary sig-nificantly from person to person and from agency to agency; the point being made here is that front-line professionals are not simply automatons who exist to carry out the will of policy makers and managers. The way a social worker manages accountability to service users may not be the same as the way they deal with accountability to the agency, and links with Du Gay's discussion regarding different 'ethical domains'.

Lipsky's focus on the mediating role of front-line professionals is significant because it points to one of the issues which he sees as central to the role of street-level bureaucrats, which is the way they exercise discretion:

Unlike lower-level workers in most organisations, street level bureaucrats have considerable discretion in determining the nature, amount and quality of benefits and sanctions provided by their agencies . . . That is not to say that street level bureaucrats are unrestrained by rules, regulations and directives from above, or by the norms and standards of their occupational group. On the contrary the major dimensions of public policy – levels of benefits, categories of eligibility, nature of rules, regulations and services – are shaped by policy elites and political and administrative officials . . . [At the same time] even public employees who do not have claims to professional status exercise considerable discretion (1980: 14).

This discretion comes about for a number of reasons. First, the range of situations which street-level bureaucrats encounter are too broad and too complex to be easily fitted into a single series of rules – there are never enough rules to cover the range of situations which front-line workers will find themselves in. Second, part of the expectation of the professional role which social workers have is not simply to respond mechanistically to what is in front of them, but to read the human and relational dimensions of a situation and devise a response accordingly. The 2011 Munro Review of Child Protection into children and families social work in the UK reinforced exactly this point in its recommendations, a key one of which was that:

Good social work practice requires forming a relationship with the child and family and using professional reasoning to judge how best to work with parents. The nature of this close engagement means that supervision, which provides the space for critical reflection, is essential for reducing the risk of errors in professionals' reasoning (Munro 2011: 11–12).

The significance of this recommendation is that while children and families social workers are expected to work within policy and guidelines and the legal framework for intervention, Professor Munro is saying that the exercise of discretion, where there is scope to do so, is equally crucial to their work.

Lipsky is, therefore, arguing that while the major parameters of policy and practice are fixed at the top level of the state, within street-level bureaucracies much front-line practice is conducted in this more indeterminate realm. It is in situations where policy and legislation offer only partial and sometimes even contradictory guidance that discretion, and the issues of ethical judgement which accompany this, come most to the fore. The following case study considers the way two social work students exercise discretion in differing ways.

Case study

Values and exercising discretion: the case of John Garson

John Garson is a young British man who has come to the attention of Social Services after contacting the duty team of a physical disability social work team, requesting help with an application for financial support from a charity which helps members of the armed forces. John is 23 years old and grew up in Local

Authority care. After leaving school with few qualifications he worked in a series of factory jobs, and frustrated with the lack of any direction or security offered by these, he decided to join the army. John liked life in the army well enough, though he found the tension of aspects of life on tours of duty in Afghanistan got to him at times, and to deal with this he started using opiate-based painkillers, which were available from army medics, as a means of relaxing. These were widely used amongst soldiers and John would not have considered his use of these to be any sort of problem. On his third tour of duty, John was severely wounded by a roadside bomb, and it was only through the quick-thinking of his fellow soldiers in getting him quickly to a field hospital that he survived at all. John is now severely disabled and due to injuries in his legs and spine is confined to a wheelchair for the rest of his life. He has been back in the UK for just over two years now; while he has had very good occupational therapy and physiotherapy, he was not offered any psychological support or counselling, nor would he have felt able to ask for this sort of help. In addition, John has become very isolated from his social networks; his former girlfriend is now in another relationship with another man with whom she has just had a child, he only ever had intermittent contact with his mother and was never close to her, and with the passage of time his former comrades in the army have stopped visiting him. John is seriously depressed and after coming off painkillers for his injuries has started drinking heavily.

John is in receipt of an army pension and disability benefits, but has got into financial problems largely through bills he left unpaid and rent arrears he failed to deal with. He was able to deal with some of the rent arrears with assistance from a charity for injured service people around six months previously, and was supported in this by a social work student who was working with the physical disability team who helped him complete the relevant paperwork and obtain the necessary independent verification of his financial difficulties. He has now come back to the same service following being threatened with court proceedings by a debt collectors following non-payment of his utility bills. Unfortunately, the charity he applied to successfully previously only allows a single application every two years unless there is a substantial deterioration in the individual's condition. Second, while John was vague about the reasons for getting into debt in the first place with the first student social worker, when John is visited this time around he takes the opportunity to talk about his difficulties, in terms of his drinking, his debts and his isolation. John makes this disclosure because he is concerned about the way his life seems to be slipping out of his control.

Questions and discussion – exercising discretion

The purpose of this exercise is to think about the way two practitioners exercise discretion in different ways. Read through the two scenarios and consider them as alternative ways of dealing with this situation.

Scenario 1: John is visited by Susan, a social work student. She is 23 and came onto the social work course with a background in working with street homeless men. On visiting John she is extremely concerned about his isolation, his drinking

▶

and his financial problems. She sees the sorting out of his finances as the beginning of a much wider programme of support for John, including support around his alcohol dependence and psychological support. While she recognises that on a strict interpretation of the criteria for the charity application he is technically ineligible, she feels they are also open to interpretation such that John could be considered again. She also sees it as significant that John has opened up to her about his wider problems and in her work with him expresses the view that clearing his debts is only the beginning of the support she feels he needs.

Scenario 2: John is visited by Wayne, a social work student. He is 32 and came onto the social work course with a background working with older people. On visiting John, he is extremely concerned about his isolation, drinking and the general chaos of his life. On looking at the charity application form he informs John straight away that he is ineligible to obtain further support from them; the question of whether the rules are open to interpretation is not something he would not see as acceptable. Wayne's approach is to try to help John deal with his debts by obtaining a low-interest loan to clear the debt. He feels this will help John to take back responsibility for his life, rather than just clearing the debts through 'another handout'. Alongside this he puts in place support for John around his alcohol dependence as well as psychological support.

Questions

1 Discuss the ethical rationales and strengths/weaknesses of these two approaches.

2 Which social work student do you think is 'more ethical', and why?

3 Think about the scope for exercising discretion that you have in your own work/placements. How do you exercise this yourself?

In summary, the question of how we understand the way a bureaucracy actually works is more complex than it may appear at first sight. What we have tried to demonstrate here is that there are a range of different approaches. We characterised Margaret Rhodes as a *pessimist,* because her emphasis is consistently on the way social workers are determined, and almost entirely negatively in her view, by the structure of the bureaucracy. Lipsky on the other hand could be seen as an *optimist,* because he emphasises the discretionary and improvisational element, noting that this exercise sometimes exists to the point of being able to work in ways that are entirely different to the intentions of those who drafted the legislation or policy.

However, rather than seeing this optimistic and pessimistic positions as alternatives to each other, it may be useful to think of them applying to different situations along a kind of 'discretion continuum' – at one end of the spectrum are social work situations in which staff have very little room to manoeuvre, while at the other end are situations in which front-line workers have considerable opportunity to do so. As well as different situations, there are also different practitioners – exemplified by the social work students Wayne and Susan in the case above – who because of their different backgrounds and experiences will understand the capacity to exercise discretion differently. This is a question that concerns values, but also concerns what sociologists call 'agency'; meaning the things people feel able to do. In this situation, agency refers to the things people are prepared to do to make the values they believe in a reality; this combination of values and agency could be seen to come together in the form of a person's political outlook. To use our example above, we could see Wayne as someone who feels the 'handout mentality' is not just unhelpful for John, but bad for society in general. In John's case he would see this as something which is preventing him from learning, or re-learning, how to be independent and take control of his situation. He is, therefore, unlikely to be interested in reinterpreting the charity guidelines. Susan, on the other hand, looks upon John as someone who has already given a huge amount, having served his country as a soldier and ended up being severely and permanently disabled in the process. As she sees it, John should be entitled to much greater support than he has received so far, and would see the fact that he has to rely on charity applications as something of an indictment of the way society treats people like him. From her perspective, the charity application is the least of what John should be entitled to.

It is in this sense that these different political understandings inform the question of what these two students are prepared to do for John, and it is in this way that discretion has these political and ethical dimensions. This brings us back to the question of the scope for discretion within bureaucratic structures, and if it is the case, as suggested at the beginning of the chapter, whether the shift towards neo-liberalism has been accompanied by an attempt to limit or alter the scope of social work's discretion, as part of a project of seeking to alter what John Clarke has called 'the meaning of welfare' (Clarke 2000: 3). It is this question that leads us to the issue about an attempt to reconstruct design and purpose of the bureaucracy – the question of managerialism.

Managerialism: end of the road for professional discretion?

We began this chapter with a discussion of the OFSTED report into children and families social work and quoted a social worker who noted that the issue of staff working extra hours 'just to keep up . . . is "hidden" due to the expectations of management and the ethos of disciplinaries. We are frightened to say that we cannot manage our workloads' (2010: 13). This personal account, which expresses something many social workers will recognise, expresses a dichotomy between the worlds of front-line social workers and management, suggesting some kind of separation between these two worlds. While this might be seen to a lesser or greater extent in all street-level bureaucracies, what we want to explore here is the idea that this division has been significantly exacerbated through the development of a particular set of ideas which have had a huge influence on the theory and practice of public management, which have become known as managerialism.

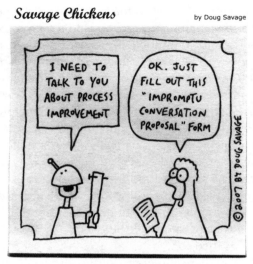

Source: Doug Savage (www.savagechickens.com)

What is managerialism? The cartoon above points to the absurdity of the convoluted forms of bureaucracy associated with it, but managerialism is more than this. Most commentators on this issue understand the emergence of managerialism in the context of the emergence of neo-liberalism in the 1980s and 1990s. Stuart Hall put this incisively when he argued that 'Managerialism is not just the hallmark of neo-liberalism, but actually the motor: if neo-liberalism is a set of ideas, how neo-liberalism then gets into the system is through managerialism' (Hall 2007: 111). In Chapter 1 we noted John Clarke's argument about the two key strands within neo-liberalism: an anti-welfarist strand and an anti-statist strand. For the anti-welfarist strand, welfare spending is seen as both unproductive, in the sense that it is 'a drain on the real economy', and undesirable, in the sense that it produces 'welfare dependency' and a 'handout mentality'. For the anti-statist element within neo-liberal thinking, the problem is excessive state involvement in what should rightly be the role of the free market, seen as the most appropriate mechanism for allocating resources, goods and services (Clarke *et al.* 2000: 2–3). While neo-liberalism began under the Thatcher/Major Conservative governments in the UK, the election of a New Labour government in 1997 under Tony Blair represented essentially a continuation of neo-liberal thinking. The concept of the 'Third Way' (see Giddens 1998), for example, was equally based on the conception of a diminished role for the state in social provision.

In terms of understanding the remaking of the welfare state, and in looking at the particular impact on the social work bureaucracy, it is important to note the way both of these different strands converge. On one hand social services agencies were seen as needing to be reduced in size and scope, but also that as an organisation, the bureaucracy needed to model itself on the practices of private sector organisations with their claims of greater efficiency. This was hugely facilitated by the privatisation and outsourcing of large areas of adult social care, where those areas of provision once run by the state were taken over by new private sector companies. The logic of this privatisation of former state-run agencies gave a huge boost to the values and attitudes embodied under managerialism, and provided further justification for the managerial revolution of changing the way people were 'expected to think and behave' within bureaucratic structures (Clarke 2000: 9). Martin Parker has sought to capture this sense of the pervasiveness of managerialism as both an ideology and a practice when he notes that it

> is increasingly articulated as a universal solution to whatever problem presents itself. Management protects us against chaos and inefficiency, management guarantees that organisations, people and machines do what they claim to do. Management is . . . a new civic religion. Even if we don't share the faith in today's management, we often seem to believe that the answer is 'better' management (2002: 2).

The key point Parker implies is the way managerialist ideas were presented as common sense – 'what works' – and thereby disavowing their ideological dimension. The elevation of managerialism to the status of what Parker ironically describes as 'a new civic religion' expresses the pervasiveness of this process. This has particular significance for social work, because managerialism was crucial to the displacement of a professionally based ethos which had previously been dominant in social work bureaucracies. Clarke notes that:

> Managerialism – like professionalism – defines a set of expectations, values and beliefs. It is a normative system concerning what counts as valuable knowledge, who knows it and who is empowered to act in what ways as a consequence. Indeed a central issue in the managerialisation of public services has been to displace or subordinate the claims of professionals. It can no longer be assumed that 'professionals know best', rather we are invited to accept that managers 'do the right thing' . . . Public service organisations have [thus] come to 'think' managerially about themselves, their 'business' and their relationships with others (2000: 9).

Managerialism in social work has thus involved the supplanting of a professionally based ethos for a managerial one. John Harris has noted that this involves a major change in the role and understanding of the social work bureaucracy:

> In the post-war welfare state, the reliance on professionalism and the assumption of citizen passivity led to state social work being provided through bureau-professional regimes in which priority was given to expert knowledge. The corollary was the subordination of citizens without expert knowledge to bureau-professional authority, in what were seen as their own interests (Harris 1999: 918).

Harris's arguments here can be linked with the discussion on the changing significance of the concept of empowerment in the previous chapter. While the old style bureau-professional regimes were characterised by state provision accompanied by professionals who 'knew best', the new style managerial regimes favour a so-called mixed economy of providers and professionals whose job it is to empower service users to look after themselves. As our previous chapter noted, this empowerment takes place in a context where the availability and eligibility for services has been significantly reduced, with significant areas of provision now run on a for-profit basis.

Other commentators have noted the way in which the rise of managerialism allows us to understand a certain irony in the way some apparently progressive agendas in social work, such as service user involvement, are being promoted. Cowden and Singh (2006) have argued, for example, that the development of this agenda needs to be seen as a sign not so much as indicative of a more enlightened attitude to service users, but more as part of an ideological battle over 'old' and 'new' conceptions of welfare. The service user agenda was one where old professional concepts of 'knowing best' were criticised as patronising, as well as insufficiently responsive to the declared aspirations of service users. Whilst there was often truth in this, the alternatives that came in the wake of community care legislation were not necessarily any better. And while the agenda around service user involvement has wide support within social work, it is at the end of the day managers who retain the capacity to decide the terms on which service users are involved, or not as the case may be (Cowden and Singh 2006).

This is of a piece with the way managerialism has become dominant through the public sector by conjuring up a world of greater transparency, accountability and flexibility for service users in opposition to an inflexible statist bureaucracy ruled over by inscrutable professionals. In spite of the pervasiveness of this image, research into these areas demonstrates that although there were many inadequacies in what went before, the introduction of market forces into social care does not necessarily lead to any of these outcomes being realised. As Malcolm Carey notes in a recent survey of state of social work:

> Within the private sector dominated market of residential and nursing home care, complex and convoluted rituals of mergers, take-overs, sales and closures have continued . . . As a consequence such markets have helped to generate unstable (and therefore potentially unsafe) living and 'support' environments for many residents. For example, recent research has highlighted how many private sector providers have failed to meet basic standards of care . . . Also recent plans by the Commission for Social Care Inspection to reduce the number of care home inspectors, including children's homes, suggests that presently unacceptable standards may fall even further (2008a: 923).

Most of the evidence for Carey's conclusions comes from government's own reports, and material such as this makes depressing reading when thinking about the ways in which bureaucratic structures limit the scope for ethical agency by social workers. In an overall sense, the response to the dominance of managerialism within the social work profession has been one of profound frustration and disorientation at the changes that have come about. This sense of fragmentation is exacerbated also by the way large sections of the social care direct provision has further declined in quality through privatisation, particularly where work is undertaken by lowly paid, lowly skilled or untrained staff. As Carey notes 'key sectors of social care are now dominated by business interests, many of which, in principle, seek to gain profits' (2008a: 919), and he goes on to note that:

> the consequences for social work practitioners have been many and have included adherence to numerous (and typically convoluted) administrative procedures and protocols, the rationalisation of social work practice, which has led to intense deskilling, and the virtual removal of therapeutic interventions and service provision (2008a: 919).

In 2006 a grouping calling itself the social work manifesto expressed the view that:

> our work is shaped by managerialism, by the fragmentation of services, by financial restrictions and lack of resources, by increased bureaucracy and workloads, by the domination of care-management approaches, with their associated performance indicators, and by the increased use of the private sector. These trends have long been present in state social work, but they now dominate the work of frontline social workers and shape the welfare services offered to clients. The effect has been to increase the distance between managers and frontline workers, and between workers and service users.

Rather than being isolated, this sense of a disjuncture between practitioners' ideas on what social work should be about and what is actually happening in reality is echoed throughout most research into the impact of managerialism on social work. In a related piece of research, where Malcolm Carey has asked front-line practitioners to describe the nature of the changes in their jobs which have been brought about by managerial practices, an equally negative picture is portrayed. One social worker, Linda, expresses these in terms of how different the job is compared to her expectation of what it would be like:

> It's just such a routine job now, and quite tedious. There's no real freedom in what you do, and everyone seems pretty fed up most of the time . . . It's just all this paper work and there's no money for services . . . I do feel terrible completing those assessment forms knowing there's no budget for anything . . . We are always hearing about new policies – 'best value' is the most recent . . . but I've seen little evidence [of positive change] . . . Nobody cares about social work (Carey 2008b: 349).

In the same article, Carey interviews another worker, Tony, who expresses a slightly more optimistic picture of his work:

> There's too much bureaucracy in the job, that's the main problem. However you can find a way around [the bureaucracy], and make time for carers and clients . . . I enjoy the work . . . There's little money about [for support services for clients] but you can still change things for some people . . . I've counselled people during assessments,

and also done a bit of group work with families, especially [informal] carers . . . You have to believe in something (2008b: 351).

These accounts both illustrate that what managerialism is managing is services run with declining resources, a fact which is denied through an obsessive emphasis on 'efficiencies'. It is this more than anything which creates the sense that people at the top fail to understand or even engage with the issues faced by social workers on the front line. The sociologist Pierre Bourdieu has argued that it is this which constitutes the 'profoundly contradictory basis of the mission' of social work under present conditions:

> Social workers must fight unceasingly on two fronts; against those they want to help and who are too demoralised to take a hand in their own interests, let alone the interests of the collectivity; on the other hand, against administrations and bureaucrats divided and enclosed in separate universes (2002: 190).

Defending bureaucracy against itself?

The question which has been addressed throughout this chapter concerns the issue of bureaucracy and ethical or moral agency – how much do bureaucratic structures suppress, undermine, facilitate or encourage ethical practice within social work. The answer is not entirely straightforward. Certain kinds of bureaucracy and bureaucratic roles undoubtedly do undermine moral agency, though it would be a mistake to see this as an inherent quality of bureaucracies. We note here the value of Paul du Gay's arguments about bureaucracy and ethics for social work, in that one of the most important ways ethical attributes may be experienced in social work, by service users at the very least, is about the way practitioners behave within a bureaucracy. To be a good bureaucrat in this sense is not about a coldly technical rationality, but rather is about an awareness of the needs of the people relying on you (2000: 4). It is in this way that Du Gay could be seen as linking the issue of behaviour within the bureaucracy with the ethics of public duty. However, it is in this sense of a focus on ethics that we can return to the point made by Bryan Turner on Weber, that it is one thing to argue for the inevitability of bureaucracy as a means of organising society, and another to endorse the rationales of the bureaucracy at any given point in time (1996: 358). This point becomes all the more pertinent in a world where the state is continuing to privatise what were once functions controlled entirely by the state, leaving those practitioners working for the state with reduced leverage to effect the change which is the very rationale for entering social work. Are social workers, therefore, destined then to remain prisoners of this particular form of neo-liberal form of bureaucracy? Pierre Bourdieu makes an insightful point when he argues that

> Paradoxically, the rigidity of bureaucratic institutions is such that, despite what Max Weber said about them, they can only function . . . thanks to the initiative, the

inventiveness, if not the charisma of those who are the least imprisoned in their function . . . And it is undoubtedly these contradictions emanating from bureaucratic divisions that open up a margin of manoeuvre, initiative and freedom which can be used by those whom, in breaking with bureaucratic routines and regulations, defend bureaucracy against itself (2002: 191).

Amongst social workers there will always be some of us who feel 'the weight of the world' more than others. But what Bourdieu offers here is the idea that just as bureaucracies are made by people, so can they be unmade by people. In this sense, our ethical duty may be best served by refusing to allow ourselves to become mentally, psychologically and practically imprisoned by the iron cage, and in doing so, we can come to realise that its bars are not as fixed as we are told they are. It is important to realise in this sense that social work only became a profession out of a form of imagined social solidarity which the welfare state represented. Through the dominance of neo-liberalism, this form of solidarity has been hollowed out and in some cases emptied altogether – yet this system itself is far from invulnerable to challenge, and it is in this process of challenge that new forms of solidarity will emerge and social work's ethical mission will again be fought over and reconstructed.

Summary

This chapter begins by considering the widely held perception that social work is a 'prisoner of bureaucracy'. We then look at the ways different writers have sought to define bureaucracy, looking again at the work of Max Weber, as well as at the way his work has been used to understand the relationship between social work and bureaucracy.

We developed a typology of approaches here based on the question of how much bureaucracy defined the actual job of the social worker, characterising Margaret Rhodes as a 'pessimist' with Michael Lipsky seen as an 'optimist'. We went on to talk about the negative impact of managerialism on social work, linking this with the discussion of neo-liberalism in Chapters 1 and 4. We concluded that this has had a hugely detrimental and demoralising effect on social work, but that this was not itself invulnerable to challenge; indeed the deployment of consciously ethical social work practice makes it a necessity that many of the manifestations of managerialism are questioned and challenged by practitioners.

Further reading

In terms of the earlier discussion about whether social workers in a bureaucracy can exert moral agency, two books by Rhodes and Lipsky have continuing resonance: Lipsky, M. (1980) *Street Level Bureaucracy: Dilemmas of the Individual in Public Service,* Russel Sage Foundation, New York; and Rhodes, M. (1991) *Ethical*

Dilemmas in Social Work Practice, Family Service America Press, Milwaukee, Wisconsin.

In terms of the contemporary situation, we recommend Carey, M. (2008) 'Everything Must Go? The Privatisation of State Social Work'. In *British Journal of Social Work* 38 (5); and Clarke, J. (2000) *New Managerialism, New Welfare,* Sage, London.

For an interesting discussion of contemporary managerialism and service-user involvement see Cowden, S. and Singh, G. (2006) 'The "User": Friend, Foe or Fetish? A Critical Exploration of User Involvement in Health and Social Care'. *Critical Social Policy,* November.

For a discussion on the impact of the idea of modernisation on social work practice we recommend Harris, J. and White, V. (2009) *Modernising Social Work: Critical Considerations,* Policy Press, Bristol.

Part 3

THEORISING ETHICAL
PRACTICE

Respect for the person, self-determination and the idea of universality: the Kantian perspective

In this chapter we will:

- Explore concepts such as respect for the person, self-determination and universality through the work of Immanuel Kant
- Illustrate how the Kantian ethical perspective can be applied to practice examples
- Discuss the contribution and the legacy of Kantian ethics on social work practice

Introduction

Respect for the person and self-determination have come to be seen as core values of social work practice, both nationally and internationally. These concepts are central to both BASW and IFSW codes of ethics and are pivotal in the various council codes of practice in England, Northern Ireland, Wales and Scotland.

Who was Immanuel Kant?

Immanuel Kant was born in Prussia in 1724. He was not from a powerful or aristocratic family; rather, his father was a labourer, and the family's financial means were very limited. He nevertheless studied mathematics, physics, philosophy and religion at the University of Königsberg at the age of 16. It was, however, only after publishing a number of unsuccessful books that Kant published his first major work on moral philosophy, entitled The *Groundwork of the Metaphysics of Morals* (1785). This publication went on to have a major influence on contemporary philosophy and established Kant as one of the most influential philosophers of all time.

This chapter begins with the exploration of social work's underlying roots in the moral philosophy of the Enlightenment. As discussed in Chapter 3, the Enlightenment was highly significant in terms of the development of philosophy and science, and was a period in which people were attempting to think about the human condition in new ways. The thoughts and ideas that developed in philosophy, politics and other sciences continue to have a major influence on contemporary society. This chapter will, therefore, examine the concepts of self-determination and human dignity through the work of an influential philosopher of the Enlightenment, Immanuel Kant. The chapter will outline key concepts in Kant's work and examine how these concepts have played such an important role in framing ideas about ethics in modern social work.

Practical reasoning and moral autonomy

For Kant, the search for and the finding of *truth* can only occur through critical examination of the reality that surrounds us through what he calls 'practical reasoning'. For example, if you have to decide whether it is right or wrong (the truth) to support a service user who wants to give a child away through adoption, you must reflect upon the situation thoroughly before making up your mind. This concept of practical reasoning may seem fairly simple to you, but is important to remember, as Chapters 3–5 outline, that your ability to practically reason will always be influenced by the wider environment in which your practice is taking place. This includes things such as the power relationships as well as the bureaucratic environment.

In addition to these, Kant also warns us that our *understanding* of the reality around us will often depend on our experiences in the world itself. Therefore, if you work with that same young woman who is experiencing an unwanted pregnancy, and who is contemplating an adoption, some of your personal experience may indeed affect your understanding of adoption. For example, if you were yourself adopted, your experience may indeed affect your understanding of adoption and termination of pregnancy (see Chapter 2 for further discussion). In Kantian terms, knowledge does not exist in a vacuum because reality is constructed through each of our various experiences in the world.

Therefore, as a starting point in Kantian theory, we must realise that 'knowledge' does not always equate with *truth,* even when you think you have found a proof which seems difficult to argue against.

What is practical reason?

Practical reason is the general human capacity for resolving through reflection the question of what one is to do (Wallace 2003).

Case study

Elliot and the gender identity disorder diagnostic

Elliot is a nine-year-old boy, who is referred by the school to his Local Authority for an assessment because of his problematic behaviour in the classroom. Elliot lives in a small town north of Coventry. He is currently in year five. During the first meeting with the social worker, the parents explain that before beginning this current academic year, Elliot had always been a 'good boy' but since November this year, he has increasingly withdrawn into himself, and has begun to pick fights with others, which got him into trouble more than once. They also explain that Elliot is increasingly struggling with academic work and that he won't accept any help from anyone when it is time to do his homework. When Elliot is asked about his social network, he says that he hates everyone at school. He explains he used to hang around a group of girls last year, but since the beginning of the school year they have started calling him names such as 'gay' and 'queer'. The boys, with whom he feels he never had any affinity, have also started to reject him even more directly than before. Elliot's parents are worried because they have observed, on a couple of occasions, little cuts on his forearms. When the social worker explores what Elliot likes to do outside school, the parents explain that he has always asked to take ballet classes, but the prices of these classes have always been too expensive for them to afford. Activities which are cheaper, like football, have never interested him. Elliot has never wanted to invite boys home, even for his birthday parties. He has never been a popular boy, but in the last year, things have got worse.

Looking back at their family history, Elliot's parents recall that he has never really been 'boisterous' and that deeply, he is more of a gentle and sensitive type of boy. He often said he would have loved to be a girl, and they recall Elliot playing with his favourite toys (his cousin's old Barbie) when he was a child. They explained that they even caught him up dressing in his mum's clothes last year but that this was too much for them to handle. They did not mind him playing with Barbies, but dressing like a girl 'was totally unacceptable'. Recalling this situation, the parents felt they had addressed this issue well since Elliot had not wished to dress as a girl again.

The social worker, who is a little puzzled about this new case, asks her supervisor, a qualified psychologist, for her thoughts on the assessment of the case. The supervisor immediately tells the social worker that she should not continue to work with Elliot, and that she should refer him in paediatric psychiatry for an assessment because she thinks Elliot's situation looks like he may have a 'gender identity disorder', a known mental disorder categorised in the DSM-4-TR. When the social worker, reflecting on her own family unit, questions this assertion, the supervisor immediately replies that the latest body of research asserts that the vast majority of gender-variant children are 'non-apparent' because they suppress their gender nonconformity as a consequence of parental and/or societal pressure (see Kennedy and Hellen 2010).

▶

> A month later, when the report from the psychiatrist comes back to the assessment team at social services, it clearly states that Elliot has been diagnosed as 'gender variant' and that they will contact the Local Authority again soon to establish an intervention plan with them.
>
> *Questions*
>
> 1 Do you feel that this diagnosis can be considered the 'truth'?
>
> 2 What makes you believe this?
>
> 3 Would you feel the same about the story if there was no indication on the diagnostic report to confirm Elliot's 'disorder'?

In many countries, the issue of gender nonconformity among children has largely been relegated to the realm of psychology, psychiatry and paediatrics: a 'health' issue diagnosed as 'gender identity disorder' in accordance with the DSM4-TR. According to the manual, gender identity disorder is marked by a preoccupation with cross-sex activities and appearance, a strong preference for cross-sex roles and a strong desire to be treated as the other sex (American Psychiatric Publishing 2010). However, as many clinicians from these health fields increasingly recognise, it is not childhood's gender nonconformity that is in itself 'the problem', but rather the lack of acceptance by society at large. For example, Ghosh (2009) explains that the 'variances' in gender should be understood as being part of a process rather than being considered as an outcome at any given time, and that many well-established social norms, such as 'boys wear trousers and girls wear skirts if they want' which tend to favour gender-conforming people, tend to cause distress and other issues among these children and their family. Furthermore, many researchers have begun to posit that gender nonconforming behaviours are only socially constructed and that they have nothing to do with personal deficiencies (Langer and Martin 2004, Else 2006) as suggested in the DSV4-TR. In Elliot's story, we have tried to show that knowledge is constructed and that the concept of *truth* in itself could be problematic, if left unquestioned. It is therefore through practical reasoning that we can begin shedding light on ethical questions. Exercising practical reasoning allows you to question different facts and/or taken-for-granted ideas in a process of reflexion and critical thinking. It is through practical reasoning that one can arrive at ethical life and what Kant calls 'moral autonomy', which is the ability to decide for one's self.

Moral autonomy, human dignity and self-determination

Kant's notion of practical reasoning is central to his theory: he believed that everyone was capable of practical reasoning. Because everyone is capable of

What is moral autonomy?

Moral autonomy is a Kantian term that means the capacity to make morally right decisions. Moral autonomy is only possible because all people have the ability for practical reasoning. In social work, this means that even when someone prescribes a rule to follow, a 'morally autonomous' person will be able to think critically and reason before deciding to apply the rule or not.

practical reasoning, that is, to think for themselves, everyone should also be considered as self-determining, and able to make decisions for themselves. Indeed, according to Kant, people should be treated with dignity because they are rational agents, that is, free agents capable of making their own decisions, setting their own goals and guiding their conduct through reason (Rachels 1986). A Kantian approach, therefore, supposes that all individuals, because they can think, should be seen as having the ability to make decisions for them, in other words, to be self-determining.

You must be wondering if practical reasoning, as understood by Kant, is really something that everyone has the ability to undertake. Because social workers intervene with different service user groups, some of which have, for example, power of attorney (that means that they cannot decide for themselves in certain or all areas of their lives), it may be legitimate to ask whether this principle can really apply to everyone.

To answer this question, it is useful to examine the social and historical contexts in which Kant lived while developing his theory. In Europe in the eighteenth century many groups of people, such as the disabled, those with limited cognitive abilities, immigrants and even women, did not have citizenship rights like men. Therefore, it is not likely that these groups were taken into consideration in Kant's original theory. In other words, when he wrote his book, Kant probably had in mind only middle-class males of German descent. However, this does not mean that groups that were not part of Kant's original understanding should be excluded from this principle. Indeed, while some groups of service users may not be legally able to make decisions for themselves in some areas of their lives, it does not mean they are unable to be self-determining in other areas. While Kant's emphasis on self-determination may not mean the same for all user groups, it is clear that all individuals have the ability to be self-determining in at least certain areas of their lives.

While we started to answer this question in part, in Chapter 5, when discussing the positive side of bureaucracy, Kant explains that the process of practical reasoning must always be undertaken in relation to three key principles:

- The intentions behind the action must be good.
- The action must be done out of a sense of duty.
- The action must be based on the 'good moral law'.

These three elements, when combined with the process of practical reasoning, will help define the morally right course of action according to Kant. We shall now examine these three principles briefly.

The principle of good intention

The first principle concerns the intention of the person in undertaking an action. We recall from the above discussion that when we are faced with a situation in social work and are required to make a decision, we must use our practical reasoning and question the different aspects of the situation to help us make that decision. However, moral autonomy and practical reasoning are not sufficient, according to Kant, for performing good actions. We also need to examine the intention behind the action, that is, 'why we want to do such and such' and ensure that the action derives from what Kant calls the 'good will', that is, that our intentions are good.

To illustrate this point, let us take the example of a social worker who usually displays good judgement in her practice. One day, she decides to bend a rule slightly to help a person who needs a particular service but does not meet the criteria. Even if the social worker was reprimanded for her action, bending the rule would still be considered the right action if the intention behind it (i.e. helping the service user) was good. On the other hand, a person may be very generous and always give money to charity. If the person does this with no other intention than to help the charity, then, for Kant, the action is morally good. However, if the person gives money to charity only for tax purposes, then the action would not be considered good in a Kantian sense because it is not performed out of good will, even if the charity still benefits from the donations.

What is the concept of good will?

A central feature of Kant's work is the idea that for an action to be good it must have been undertaken on the basis of good will and good intentions. If this is the case, then the action can be considered good, regardless of the consequences that result from it.

Therefore, what constitutes goodness should not simply be evaluated on the basis of the result of an action. Instead, a Kantian approach examines the basis of the intention or motivation behind the action in order to decide if an action is morally right or wrong. Therefore, according to Kant, it does not matter how many good qualities a person has: if the intention behind the action is wrong, then the action cannot be morally right.

The Milgram experiment is a good example of this principle. In this experiment, conducted in the 1960s, Stanley Milgram, then researcher at Yale University, wanted to examine how people responded to authority. He asked a number of participants to administer an electric shock (simulated) to another person whom they could not see, every time that person responded incorrectly to a question. Most participants, though feeling quite uncomfortable, administered the electric shock because they were asked to by a man in a white coat. Since this was only an experiment, the electric shocks were not real, and nobody in the experiment was actually hurt. Now, even though this was the case, does this make the participants' actions right? We must remind ourselves that the participants were only acting out of respect for authority. Though it seems obvious in this example, it is very likely that Kant would say that the actions were morally wrong. The actions would not be considered good because the intention behind the actions was not good. While we all agree that it would be hardly possible to find a good intention behind administering an electric shock to someone, what is important to note here is that it is really the *intention* behind the action that counts and not the consequence of the action itself. Indeed, Kant believes in the assertion that nothing is unconditionally good except good will. It is, therefore, the intention behind the action that matters, not the action itself. Thus, for Kant it is the intention, rather than the consequences, that is crucial, even though, and unfortunately so, the good intention may not result in good consequences. To remind ourselves of this point in a single phrase, in Kantian ethics, 'the end never justifies the means'. In other words, the consequences of an action, though positive in the end, can never be justified by an action that is not well intentioned.

The principle of duty

We have seen thus far that the morally right action, or in the case of social work, an ethical intervention or decision reflecting Kantian principles, is an

What is a duty?

A duty is something that someone ought to do and implies a moral obligation. For example, duties in social work are usually articulated not only within codes of ethics and codes of practice, but also within certain laws.

action that involves thought and questioning through practical reasoning; it is undertaken out of good intentions or, as Kant calls it, out of good will. The ethical social worker will therefore be called upon to challenge the many assumptions that are likely to be observed in practice, will refuse to take anything for granted and will do so for the right reasons.

This brings us to a discussion regarding another important concept in Kantian ethics, that of 'duty'. Kant tells us that every action must also be undertaken out of a sense of duty. 'Duty to what?' we might ask. Let us have a look at the concept of duties, in the context of social work.

For social work, action out of duty means following what is in your code of ethics, as long as you do not take the latter's contents for granted and always commit yourself to thinking it through by carefully examining its application to different situations through practical reasoning. The concept of duty is therefore important and relates, in this regard, to the principles of ethical practice set out in the code of ethics of the British Association of Social Workers (BASW), for example (2002: 2). According to this code, the first duty of social workers is to respect basic human rights as expressed in the United Nations *Universal Declaration of Human Rights* and other international conventions derived from it. Five other principles that emphasise the value base of social work are then outlined. We shall return to some of these principles later in this chapter. For the moment, we can observe that the BASW code of ethics is formulated around different duties that are relevant to the profession. In this sense, we can therefore talk about a duty-based ethics.

However, we discussed earlier that in a Kantian sense, behaving a certain way out of pure social conformity or in response to authority, for example, does not necessarily indicate a good action. In other words, doing something because we have been conditioned to do so is not right, even though we may have been told that it is. Furthermore, Kant reasoned that setting out to do the right thing because one feels 'happy' to do so is not as worthy doing the right thing because one feels a moral obligation to do so and rationally thought about the action beforehand (the notion of intention). So how do we know that what is in the code of ethics is really 'the duty' we should undertake as a social worker? We may see here a paradox in interpreting Kant's moral theory. On the one hand, Kant tells us not to take anything for granted and always use practical reasoning in examining evidence. On the other hand, he also tells us that we ought to act out of a sense of duty to moral law. Can we just apply codes of ethics in social work to any situation? Where does this leave us? What if a duty conflicts with another one? For example, what if a social worker is faced with a situation whereby she has the duty to protect someone from harm, at the same time than enabling them to make their own decisions? In order to shed some light on this aspect of duty, we shall have to look at what, according to Kant, is good moral law.

Defining and using good moral law, or commands

For Kant, to live according to a sense of duty, as described above, is to live an ethical life. Ethical life does not depend on our feeling of rightness or wrongness, but instead on our pursuit of practical reason. To do so, we must think about our sense of duty as being formulated around *'moral laws'* that Kant believed were essential to ethical life. However, we may wonder if a certain incompatibility exists between, on the one hand, Kant's arguments in favour of practical reasoning and, on the other hand, his insistence on adhering to moral laws. The answer to this lies in the way Kant understands the concept of moral law. Moral laws, according to Kant, are not rules that directly influence actions; rather, they put in place the principles that allow people to act out of good will and out of a sense of duty, while at the same time using their ability for practical reasoning. These principles, in Kant's theory, refer to that of 'imperative' or *rules to adhere to*, as we shall refer to it in this book.

Kant considered two basic types of rules: the *hypothetical rule* and the *categorical rule*. Hypothetical rules *advise* you on a course of action, but that generally implies a condition, meaning that it is usually formulated using an 'if' and 'then' structure. For example, a hypothetical rule might be something along the lines of 'if you want to be a good citizen, then exercise your right to vote'. This example stresses the conditional aspect of good citizenship through voting. It also stress that if you do not want to be a good citizen, you do not need to vote. It is therefore conditional in nature.

A categorical rule, on the other hand, is a rule that instructs people what to do regardless of the reason or without reference to any other end (Kant 1785). For example, a categorical rule might be 'always participate fully in society'. This is a categorical rule because it proposes a direction that must be followed regardless of the possible outcome. In this case, it would include voting, but does not exclude other forms of citizenship participation like volunteering, for example. For Kant, categorical rules are central to the articulation of good moral laws because, unlike the hypothetical one, it is not a means to something else; as you will remember, good actions in Kantian morality must be undertaken because they are right in themselves, rather than as a means to an end.

What is a moral law?

A moral law is a principle that is defined by the person who is making a decision, through practical reasoning. The articulation of the moral law should always respect two basic conditions or principles:

It must underpin a *fundamental respect for the person*, and you must be able to make it *universal to all*.

For Kant, it is the categorical rule that people must follow to lead an ethical life, because it is the only command that does not involve a means to an end.

To illustrate the difference between hypothetical and categorical commands, consider the following example from social work practice.

Imagine you are about to leave the office at 5 p.m. when a service user, who appears extremely distressed, arrives. Your manager asks you if you would be good enough to stay a little longer to deal with the situation. Let us imagine that you decide to stay on and help. What is your reason for doing so? You may decide to stay on and help the service user because you want to impress your manager with your dedication, which would be looked upon positively in the event of a promotion or salary increase. You may also decide to see the service user because you would feel guilty if you did not, that something might happen to her and you would feel responsible. Alternatively, you may accept to see the service user simply because she is distressed and in need of help, even though you were about to leave the office. In other words, you may see her out of respect for her as a person. The first two reasons for agreeing to see the service user are based on Kant's *hypothetical rules* because the service user is merely seen as a means to an end, whether for your own self-interest in gaining a promotion or for avoiding your own feelings of guilt (if you want a promotion, you must work harder, if you want to have good appraisal, you must see the service user). On the other hand, seeing the service user simply because she is distressed and needs help, even though it may be inconvenient for you, represents a *categorical rule*; your motive for seeing the service user is not based on any other end than to respond to her need, and in this sense you are acting solely out of a sense of moral duty.

However, how can a person be sure that a rule, even if it is categorical, will lead to ethical life? Kant defines two principles in which the rule must fit:

• It must always be based on the respect for the person.

• It must always be universal, that is, applicable in all situations.

Respect for the person

'Respect for persons' is a principle that presupposes that the rule should never use another person as a means to an end. This is consistent with the concepts of good will and paying little attention to consequences discussed above. This principle tells us that a person should never be treated as a means to an end, but must always be treated as an end in itself. To understand this, consider again the example of the manager who asks you to stay at work later than usual to see a service user who is distressed and needs immediate attention. A categorical rule for this example would be 'always help people who are in need'. If you applied this command to the situation, then you would either see the service user right away or you would arrange for an alternative solution so that she could eventually get the help she needed. Helping someone only because one wants to impress others would not be acting in accordance with respect for that person and constitutes treating them as a means to an end.

Universality

Universality, for Kant, is principle that determines a right action on the basis that if it is right for one, it is right for all, and may thus be adopted as a 'universal law'. This means that whatever you intend to do, you must make sure that your action would be ethical regardless of the context in which it takes place and could thus be universalised. This categorical rule therefore emphasises that a good action will be good to whomever, wherever and whenever. Again, the command given in the example of the social worker, that is, questioning herself about staying or not to help the distressed service user, would clearly meet the universality criteria, as whatever situation, a person would be happy to be on the receiving end and get help with their situation. In line with the social work duties discussed above, you can also see that when combined, they form an interesting way of 'universalising' good social work practice.

As you can see, the commands that are emerging as part of the practical reasoning process are not ready-made rules that we pick and choose whenever we need to make a decision. Instead, they give an orientation to the development of the rule that can be applied to a given situation. Combined with the notion of good intention and developed through the process of practical reasoning, these two principles (respect for the person and universality) ensure that the rule you define in a given situation will lead to the right action. We shall now examine each of these categorical commands before drawing conclusions about Kantian ethics and considering how such an approach may help in the analysis of ethical dilemmas in practice.

Summary: Moral autonomy, human dignity and self-determinative

For Kant, an ethical life is possible because people have the ability for practical reasoning and are therefore morally autonomous. Because of this quality, people who are acting out of good will and out of a sense of duty to the moral law are able to perform morally right actions. It is through the ability to reflect and think critically that a person can assess whether or not an action is ethical. To do

Reflection break

Recounting the principles of Kantian ethics:

1 Summarise what you consider to be the main points of Kant's ethical theory.

2 How might these principles be used in social work practice?

so, the person will formulate rules that will guide them in making their decision. These rules, called categorical imperatives, must be taking into consideration two principles: 'respect for the person' and 'universality'. Kant believes it is by combining these elements that all people can live an ethical life.

The following sections will examine the Kantian ethics, philosophy and principles we discussed above through the use of a social work case study.

Case study

Mark's story

Gabriella is a 27-year-old woman from Spain. She came to the UK a little more than four years ago to work. One night, when she was returning home from work, she was attacked and raped by a group of men. Despite an extensive investigation, the police were never able to find the perpetrators of this crime. Shortly after the incident, Gabriella started to suffer from depression; at the same time, she discovered she was pregnant as a result of the rape. Because of her religious beliefs, Gabriella felt she had no choice but to continue with the pregnancy, and she gave birth to Juanita three years ago. Gabriella asserts that without her religious beliefs, she would 'never have made it up to now'.

Following the birth of her daughter, Gabriella had been in touch with mental health services because her problems with depression worsened. It was noted that she had not responded significantly to either medication or the work undertaken by the community psychiatric nurse and psychologist. Things deteriorated for Gabriella when Juanita was 20 months old: Gabriella was sectioned under the 1983 Mental Health Act. While her mother was in the psychiatric hospital, Juanita was placed temporarily in foster care. Gabriella remains isolated. She has no family in the UK, has very few friends, and feels unable to return to Spain. Since she was sectioned under the Mental Health Act, Gabriella has been in and out of psychiatric hospitals and has found it increasingly difficult to care for Juanita. Realising she could no longer cope, in the last month, Gabriella gave parental consent for Juanita to be adopted under Section 47.2(a).

Justina and Mary have been in a relationship for seven years and have lived together for five years. Justina is originally from Portugal but has been living in the UK since she left university 10 years ago. Mary is British. Mary was raised as a Catholic but is not particularly religious. Justina is also Catholic and is fully involved in her local Catholic church. The couple attend church together at Christmas and Easter. For some time now, Justina and Mary have felt the desire to have a child. After carefully exploring the different options, they decided that adopting a child, as opposed to sperm donation, would be the best choice for them. They felt that this would be a more equal solution because neither woman would be the birth mother; at the same time, they would both be 'helping a child'. Justina and Mary have been on a waiting list for nearly two years, and no child has been matched with them so far.

One morning, Justina receives a phone call from their social worker at the local agency they are registered with. The social worker, Mark, explains that a mother has given her consent for her three-year-old daughter to be adopted. Since the daughter is of Spanish origin, Justina and Mary are keen on the idea of adopting the toddler. When the social worker explains to Gabriella that she has found potential parents, Gabriella is very happy, that is, until she discovers that the adopting couple are lesbians. She then becomes adamant about her daughter being adopted by a Roman Catholic family and that it is against her religion for her daughter to be raised by a same-sex couple. She insists that she wants a married heterosexual couple, 'who will be able to raise her daughter in the values she dearly believes in'. She threatens to withdraw her consent for the adoption if Social Services proceeds with Justina and Mary as the adoptive parents.

Questions

Looking back through the case study:

1 Identify the ethical dilemma facing Mark.

2 Identify the various courses of action Mark could take.

3 Write down what you feel are the most important elements to take into consideration in each course of action you identified above. Why do you feel they are important?

4 How would you express the issues facing Mark in terms of Kantian ethics?

Analysing the ethical dilemmas from a Kantian perspective

The dilemma facing Mark in the above case study raises many difficult issues regarding individual rights, welfare, self-determination and autonomy, as well as discrimination against all or some of the individuals involved.

A Kantian approach may be helpful in casting light on these issues. We now propose to look at the case study and to apply Kantian principles to the various aspects of the situation discussed above. As mentioned before, Kantian ethics focuses on a person's ability to engage in practical reasoning, the motivation and sense of duty behind an action and whether the action is compatible with good moral law in terms of it adhering to the two principles of respect for the person and universality.

How do these elements relate to the situation facing Mark in this case study? The focus of the analysis will be on the social worker, Mark, and his actions, rather than on the issues facing Gabriella, Justina and Mary, since it ultimately falls upon Mark to decide the course of action to take. After the analysis of Mark's situation through Kantian principles, we will pose some further questions and then examine the possible courses of action. We shall conclude this chapter by looking at various codes of ethics and practice in relation to Kantian ethics and then discuss the possible challenges that emerge in practice.

In order to examine the situation facing Mark and to analyse it in light of Kantian principle, we must, as with any ethical dilemma, first identify precisely what the dilemma is. There are many perspectives in which this dilemma could be analysed, but we will now focus the analysis on the dilemma as being articulated as a conflict of values between the right of self-determination of Gabriella as Juanita's birth mother relinquishing her child and the possible discrimination toward Justina and Mary as a same-sex couple wishing to adopt. Mark could take the following courses of action:

1 Let Justina and Mary know that the placement is not viable and that he will be in touch with them soon when another suitable child becomes available. In this way, Gabriella does not revoke her parental consent for Juanita to be adopted under Section 47.2(a). However, Mary and Justina are discriminated against on the basis of their sexual orientation.

2 Continue with the adoption process and undertake all necessary procedures with Justina and Mary, but at the same time run the risk of Gabriella revoking her parental consent for Juanita's adoption. If this were to occur, Juanita would likely be placed in temporary foster care until an adoption order was obtained from the court and new suitable adoptive parents were found.

This situation illustrates the nature of Mark's ethical dilemma in that he now has to make a decision one way or the other. While you may hold your own views about the best decision, it is clear that there are significant problems regarding either course of action.

Mark's moral autonomy

In what sense can a Kantian ethical framework help us resolve this dilemma? In this light, the first point is that Mark is capable of moral autonomy. Indeed, according to Kant, all individuals should be perceived as having moral autonomy, that is, that they are capable of deciding for themselves, or self-determining. They are able to make their own decisions because they are able to think. Mark received a degree in social work and is therefore capable, one assumes, of critical and independent thought. Mark is also registered as a social worker with the General Social Care Council, and as such, he must adhere to the National Occupational Standards for social work. In England, for example, it is clear that a qualified social worker must possess a certain level of 'critical thinking' in their practice:

> Think critically about their own practice in the context of the GSCC Codes of Practice, national and international codes of professional ethics and the principles of diversity and equality and social inclusion in a wide range of situations, including those associated with inter-agency and inter-professional work (National Occupational Standards for social work, cited in Brown and Rutter 2006: 1).

We therefore assume that Mark has an ability for practical reasoning with regard to this situation, as well as a good level of moral autonomy.

Mark's motivation and good will in making a decision

If we continue with the application of the Kantian perspective to resolve this ethical dilemma, the other element to examine is Mark's motivation in acting in this particular situation. Again, one can only make assumptions with regard to Mark's motivation. When the time comes for you to face an ethical dilemma in practice, it will be very important for you to have some real insight into your inclination to act in a certain way and to examine your motivations for acting carefully. As we explained above, only good motives can justify a good action in a Kantian sense.

Therefore, only the person making the decision can truly have this insight. With regard to the case study, only Mark or the social worker facing such a dilemma is able to examine their deepest motivations in acting one way or another. This is the very basis of being able to engage in critical reflection with regard to an ethical dilemma. You should therefore ask yourself the following questions: why am I inclined to act in such a way? What are my motives behind my chosen course of action? Am I *free* to act in this particular way? If not, do I have sufficient moral autonomy to challenge my own decision? Am I about to undertake this action out of a sense of duty? You must ask yourself such questions when faced with an ethical dilemma using a Kantian framework for ethical reasoning. In order to answer the questions in Mark's situation, we must also decide who is the central focus: Justina and Mary, Gabriella and Juanita, or both parties.

In order to analyse Mark's motivation in this case, we will again make some assertions and base our reasoning on Mark's commitment to the profession and his respect for the Care Council's code of practice.

We can assume that as a social worker, Mark is committed to a set of values common to social work practice. As discussed in the introduction to this section, three social work values tend to appear in the literature on social work ethics, namely, respect for persons and the self-determination of service users, commitment to the promotion of social justice and the concept of 'professional integrity' (Banks 2006: 44–6). Therefore, we can assume that Mark's inner motivation for practicing social work is compatible with these core values and the various codes of conduct and ethics.

In examining the GSCC (2002) code of practice, a relatively large number of articles may be pertinent to Mark's situation. However, our purpose here is not to name them all, but instead to focus on those that we feel are particularly relevant to motivation in this case. First, Mark has the duty to treat each person as an individual (Article 1.1 GSCC 2002) to respect and, where appropriate, to promote the individual views and wishes of all service users and carers (Article 1.2 GSCC 2002). This could be illustrated by his wish to work with both Mary/Justina and Gabrielle/Juanita. Mark must also honour his work commitments, agreements and arrangements, and when it is not possible to do so, explain the reason to service users and carers (Article 2.5 GSCC 2002). Mark must also use established procedures and processes to challenge and report dangerous, abusive, discriminatory, or exploitative behaviours and practices (Article 3.2 GSCC 2002) and avoid discriminating unlawfully or unjustifiably against service users, carers or colleagues (Article 5.5 GSCC 2002). Finally, Mark has the duty to work according to relevant standards of practice and in a lawful, safe and effective way (Article 6.1 GSCC 2002). According to the BASW (2002) code of ethics, Mark should also place service users' needs and interests before his own beliefs, aims and views, and not use professional relationships to gain personal, material or financial advantage (BASW 2002: 5). Therefore, in assuming that Mark is a qualified social worker who builds his practice around these core values and respects the above codes of practice and ethics, we may assert that Mark's motivation in this situation is to undertake social work practice within the boundaries of his profession and to leave aside any personal values he may hold. We could also posit that his motives are good because he would like to help Justina and Mary achieve their goal of adopting a child and to assist Gabriella in the adoption process in order to find a suitable and permanent placement for Juanita.

Acting out of a sense of duty: examining the situation through the categorical rules

As we have seen, Kant asserts that in order to act ethically, a person must act out of a sense of duty to good moral law, as formulated through categorical rules. We will now examine Mark's dilemma from this perspective.

Course of action 1 – the placement is deemed unviable

We begin with the first possible course of action described above, in which Mark informs Justina and Mary that the placement is not viable and that he will be contacting them again soon when another suitable child becomes available. In this way, Gabriella does not revoke her parental consent for Juanita to be adopted under Section 47.2(a), and other potential adoptive parents can be found.

This course of action would emphasise the importance of promoting and respecting the views and wishes of Gabriella. One could claim that this course of action takes into consideration the wishes of all parties, since Justina and Mary could have another child proposed to them quickly, and Gabriella could have her views taken into consideration fully. We must now examine this situation through the categorical rules. To facilitate the process of practical reasoning and to understand the difference between categorical and hypothetical rules, we will begin by providing an example of both types of rules, hypothetical and categorical. We will then examine this course of action more carefully through the principles of universality and respect for the person.

Many rules could be formulated with regard to this dilemma, as long as the rule remains general in nature. We could, for example, begin with the hypothetical rule that 'If you want to ensure the best outcome for a person in an intervention, you must do anything in your power to achieve it.' However, as we discussed above, Kant believes that a categorical rule will always result in a person being treated as a means to an end (respect for the person) and therefore, a hypothetical rule here is not satisfactory. Indeed, acting on this hypothetical rule would suppose that for the sake of the child, you are ready to use other people as a means to an end, that is, Justina and Mary. Justina and Mary's desire to have a child has been voiced for several years now, and acting in this manner would be disrespectful to them. We may wonder, however, if this hypothetical rule fails by the mere fact that it is hypothetical. Would it still fail if we articulated a categorical rule? We shall now turn to this question.

A categorical rule would therefore be 'Always put the best interests of the person you are working with first.' We must now examine this categorical rule further and test it against the principles of universality and respect for the person set out by Kant. With regard to the former, we must enquire as to whether we could render this rule universal. In other words, are there situations in which we would not want such a moral law to be universal, or could it pass the test of applicability to any situation or context? Would it be possible to find situations in which it is not justifiable to act in such a way as to put a child's interests first? Would it be acceptable, for example, to lie in order to put the interests of a person we are working with first? If it is acceptable in one situation, can we justify that lying is something that we can render universal in order to protect the interests of all service users with whom we will work in the future? Kant would certainly tell us that if everyone lied, for whatever reason, then society could not function, and the notion of trustworthiness would disappear completely. Therefore, in light of this rule, we could assert that lying would not meet the principle of universality because there are situations in which it would be morally wrong to do whatever is needed to uphold the best interests of a person with whom we are working. The end would justify the means, and this is not morally acceptable in Kantian ethics because it does not respect the person intrinsically. Therefore, we need to find a categorical rule that would satisfy both principles. To formulate such a rule, we shall now turn to the other course of action and examine it through another set of commands.

Course of action 2 – to continue with the adoption process

The second course of action is for Mark to continue with the process of working with Justina and Mary regardless of Gabriella's course of action. From Justina and Mary's point of view, this course of action would emphasise the importance of non-discriminatory and non-oppressive practice, without taking into consideration possible outcomes, even negative ones (i.e. Gabriella removing her parental consent). With regard to Mark's motivation, we mentioned earlier the importance of clearly identifying the main client. In reality, the categorical rule you use to help resolve a situation should apply to all situations and should not account for the possible consequences of the action. This is because Kantian ethics reminds us that 'what is good for one is good for all', but also that a means should not justify an end. In this sense, a categorical command that may apply to this possible course of action would be 'You should never discriminate against another person.'

The next question to ask is whether this command would satisfy the universality principle. Would it be possible to have an example in which discrimination was acceptable and necessary? Would positive discrimination be acceptable, for example? The answer to this is probably yes. For example, would it be acceptable for an agency providing services to ethnic minority women who have experienced domestic violence to positively discriminate in their recruitment strategy in order to appoint a new member who could relate to the main client group? Would this still not count as discrimination? Would our categorical command still satisfy the universality criterion? Or do we only need to formulate it better? Would our command be more universal if we refined it and specified the type of discrimination? The categorical command 'You should never discriminate negatively against a person' would probably satisfy the universality criterion since, if discrimination were accepted broadly in society, this same society would go against the principles of human rights. Therefore, the categorical rule would meet this first principle.

Would it also meet the principle of respect for the person? Recall what Kant has to say about this: 'Act so that you treat humanity, whether in your own person or that of another, always as an end and never as a means only' (Kant 1785). This principle tells us that people should never be treated as a means to an end, but always as an end in themselves. Discriminating negatively against people because of their sexual orientation would not be treating them as an end in itself, but instead, as a means to an end. Furthermore, this categorical command would also meet the principle of respect for the person. Thus, in this situation, 'never discriminate negatively against a person' would be a good moral command to follow. It would also echo, as examined earlier, our duty as social workers to respect basic human rights as set out in the United Nations *Universal Declaration of Human Rights*, which specifically asserts in Article 2:

> Everyone is entitled to all the rights and freedoms set forth in this Declaration, without distinction of any kind, such as race, colour, sex, language, religion, political or other opinion, national or social origin, property, birth or other status. Furthermore, no distinction shall be made on the basis of the political, jurisdictional, or international status of the country or territory to which a person belongs, whether it be independent, trust, non-self-governing or under any other limitation of sovereignty (United Nations 1948).

Applied to the case above, this would probably result in Mark deciding to continue his work with Justina and Mary in order not to discriminate against them, even though Gabriella is likely to retract her voluntary agreement for the adoption and the process may take longer.

Reflection break

Looking through your code of practice, identify which elements would help Mark resolve the ethical dilemma presented in the case study.

1 Which of these elements becomes apparent in terms of Kantian principles?
2 How do they help in a course of action that stresses the importance of self-determination, duty and autonomy?

This is one possible way of managing the ethical dilemma applying a Kantian approach. You may find the solution acceptable, or perhaps you could think of another categorical rule to test in this particular dilemma. What is important in Kantian ethics is to use your practical reason in examining your motivation for acting, and to always intervene out of a sense of duty, that is, by formulating rules that meet the two principles of universality and respect for the person, and which is coherent with your professional duties, that is those articulated in various codes of ethics in social work. If the categorical rule satisfies the two principles of universality and respect for the person, and your motivations are good in the intervention, then it is very likely that your decision is Kantian in essence.

You may realise that many articles found in the codes of ethics (BASW) and the code of conduct (GSCC) are Kantian in nature. This Kantian legacy has a

Reflection break

Biestek, a Christian priest doing social work, had already articulated the following principles for social work:

- Individualisation
- Purpose expression of feelings
- Controlled emotional involvement
- Acceptance
- Non-judgemental attitude
- Client self-determination
- Confidentiality

(Biestek 1961)

1 What link can you make between these principles and the Kantian approach to ethics discussed above?
2 Do you feel they are adequate to social work contemporary practice?
3 What are the weaknesses of such principles?

long history in social work, with literature on social work from the 1960s already articulating social work principles around Kantian principles.

The principles articulated by Biestek are mostly Kantian in nature since they are all underpinned by the respect for the person and human dignity and worth. Having said that, to be truly in a Kantian perspective, these principles would need to be articulated in commands that meet the criteria of respect for the person and universality, as we saw above, be subjected to the notion of practical reasoning, and the action be undertaken out of good will.

We have demonstrated that practical reasoning as a way of weighing different courses of action based on Kantian principles is useful in managing ethical dilemmas. Of course, in practice, social workers must adhere to the various laws, policies, guidelines and procedures of their agencies and governments, not to mention all the practical pressures that social workers must face on a daily basis! Such factors can affect the application of the Kantian approach in practice, a point which Banks (1995) notes when she states that the interpretation of Kant's moral philosophy may pose a problem for practical ethics because principles of self-determination and confidentiality often clash with existing rules and regulations. Warburton (1999) additionally argues that Kant's moral principles do not always yield satisfactory solutions to moral questions. For example, the Adoption and Children Act 2002 states that the paramount consideration of the court must be the child's welfare. The court or adoption agency must at all times bear in mind that, in general, a delay in coming to a decision is likely to prejudice the child's welfare (1.2; 1.3). Also to be considered in situations such as Justina and Mary's is the Equality Act (Sexual Orientation) Regulations 2007, which makes it unlawful for providers of services, goods or facilities, including adoption agencies, to discriminate against their service users on the grounds of sexual orientation.

Therefore, when applying the different Kantian principles, it is important to take these laws and regulation into consideration and not only reason in terms of Kantian principles, as demonstrated above. However, from a Kantian perspective, you should not take for granted all the rules and regulations that are imposed on you, but instead reason practically and examine such rules and regulations before applying them to your ethical dilemma. A Kantian perspective is therefore helpful in managing the dilemma, but it cannot be applied without careful thought. You should be ready to challenge, if appropriate, any law or regulation that would be detrimental to a service user, if such a challenge follows Kantian ethics. Thus it is not simply about applying Kantian principles for the sake of applying them, but about using these principles to help us better understand how to approach the dilemmas that occur in day-to-day practice. As Warburton illustrates, Kantian principles may appear impractical in some situations:

> If, for example, I have a duty always to tell the truth, and also a duty to protect my
> friend, Kant's theory would not show me what I ought to do when these two duties

conflict. If a madman carrying an axe asked me where my friend was, my first inclination would be to tell him a lie. To tell the truth would be to shirk the duty I have to protect my friend. But on the other hand, according to Kant, to tell a lie, even in such an extreme situation, would be an immoral act: I have an absolute duty never to lie (Warburton 1999: 47).

In terms of ethical social care practice, Rhodes (1986) tells us that a Kantian legacy would imply that social workers should seek the respect of the person. However, because a Kantian approach is based on the ability to reason practically, it is important not to merely apply this principle for the sake of applying it. Using Mark's story as an example, we demonstrated that the Kantian way of resolving the ethical dilemma was not simply to apply the principle of user self-determination in an outright manner, but instead, to carefully think the case through, and examine the various principles underpinning Kantian theory. In practice, we must also balance the various interests of all the parties involved. We demonstrated in the case study that disallowing Justina and Mary to proceed with the adoption may have shown concern for Gabriella's self-determination but would not have passed the test of universality, nor would it have treated the service users as ends in themselves. Kantian ethics is also useful in that it heightens our awareness of our own self-interest in the particular situations in which we find ourselves (Vardy and Grosch 1999: 57–8) and emphasises questions of fairness. As Hugman points out, 'Kant's categorical command can be seen as a statement that implies fairness as a moral good, because it asserts that what applies for one person should apply for everyone in similar circumstances' (2005: 16). However, even though a Kantian perspective may be applied to a dilemma in practice, it is also important to remember that the situation remains a dilemma and ultimately involves the difficult task of making a decision one way or another. The Kantian perspective will, however, provide you with a framework for analysing your dilemma that is compatible with the values of social work as formulated in our codes of practice, in other words, a commitment to the values of an individual's right to dignity, respect, privacy and confidentiality. These values are directly inspired by Kant's moral philosophy and remain important in everyday social work practice.

Summary

Kant was one of the most important moral philosophers of the Enlightenment, and his philosophy continues to have a major influence on contemporary moral theory and attitudes, not the least of which is contemporary social work practice. Kant based his moral philosophy on the fact that all human beings have the ability to reason, and that as long as actions are taken out of good will and a sense of duty, they are morally right. For Kant, a good moral law must meet the criteria of two categorical commands: universality and respect for the person. The influence of the Kantian tradition on social work today is illustrated by the various codes of ethics and practice that exist in the profession and which are based on the principles of respect for the person and the notion that 'what is good for one is also good for all'.

Further reading

If you want to further your reading on Kantian ethics, this book will take you into very informative discussions about the various aspects of this moral theory: Wood, A. (2008) *Kantian Ethics,* Cambridge University Press, New York. While not specifically written for a social work audience, it nevertheless provides some interesting applications of Kantian theory to contemporary social problems.

Hill, T. E. J. (ed.) (2009) *The Blackwell Guide to Kant's Ethics,* Blackwell, Chichester. This authoritative guide provides in-depth explanations as well as new perspectives on Kant's most important contribution to ethics, *The Groundwork for Metaphysics of Morals (1785) and The Metaphysics of Morals (1798).* While this collection of texts presents many complex ideas, it is nevertheless written in an accessible manner.

CHAPTER 7

Social justice: the ethics of Mill and Rawls

Chapter outline

In this chapter we will:

- Explore the concept of social justice, a core value of social work, through the work of John Stuart Mill and John Rawls
- Illustrate the way their theories can assist in understanding an ethical issue related to social justice
- Discuss the strengths and weaknesses of both approaches as applied to social work practice

Introduction

Social justice is the second core principle of social work which we will be discussing in this book. It appears as such in the IFSW and BASW codes of ethics and serves, along with the principle of human dignity, as a central motivation and justification for social work action (IFSW 2000). The term 'justice' itself is very broad and can be understood differently depending on the many theoretical frameworks applied to it. In fact, like the concept of power discussed in Chapter 3, Marshall (1998) notes that the concept of social justice is subject to wide disagreement among sociologists, social psychologists and philosophers. In the context of this book, the concept of social justice broadly relates to justice applied to social life. However, what does the term justice mean? What does it imply? How can we ensure that we are acting in a social justice perspective? How can we make the right decisions when faced with a dilemma that brings to light issues of social justice?

Before answering these questions, we shall examine, in this chapter, two sets of theories that provide us with a framework for understanding the concept of justice. Exploring these two theoretical perspectives will not only allow us to better understand what is required for a just outcome, but will also provide us with a framework for analysing specific situations in social work practice and for applying these perspectives more generally to social life.

There are many theories about the concept of justice that we could have examined in this chapter. Although the choice was not any easy one, we decided on two ethical theories that we believe are relevant to social work practice and comprise principles of justice that are pertinent to social work. The first is Mill's Utilitarian ethics. We chose this theory because the principles it outlines concern mostly social issues. The principles, in turn, affect social work practice indirectly through the way social welfare is organised. The second theory we have decided to include in this chapter is Rawls's theory of justice. Rawls remains one of the most influential philosophers of our time. Justice, as formulated by Rawls, is also relevant to social work because it forms the basis of many laws and policies, especially those of liberal orientations.

Both theories will be helpful in developing our understanding of justice and provide us with two ethical theories that can be used for decision-making purposes in dilemmas related to social work ethics.

The case study central to this chapter concerns a social worker who is faced with a dilemma involving the assessment of a young asylum seeker who presents herself as a minor; issues emerge with regard to age identification and resource allocation. As in the previous chapters, we will then analyse the situation in the light of Utilitarian principles and Rawls's theory of justice and establish links with the principle of social justice as formulated in IFSW, BASW and GSCC codes. The purpose here is to help develop your understanding of the continued influence of these theories on the formulation and management of ethical issues in social work and to assist you in the process of practical reasoning. We will conclude this chapter by drawing some conclusions about the meaning of social justice as applied to contemporary social work.

Utilitarian ethics

Utilitarianism is often described as a form of *ethical consequentialism*. This means that in order to assess an action as being right or wrong in a given situation, we must look at the consequences of applying that action.

For example, if you had to make a decision to give money or not to a homeless person on the street, you could justify your action by looking at it from different perspectives. First, you could say that giving money to a homeless person is the right thing to do because you have been lucky in life, you have a home and enough money to survive, and therefore you should help others by sharing what you have. This would not be a consequentialist way of looking at a situation because instead of looking at the consequence of giving money or not to a homeless person, you are looking at your motivation for acting or not. You will remember that this way of managing decisions was covered in the last chapter and belongs to a more Kantian form of ethics, in which the motivation behind the action is central (see Chapter 6 for further details). If you were to adopt a consequentialist perspective, you would instead think about all the possible consequences that giving money or not may bring for the various parties involved. Far from being exhaustive in terms of consequences, you could think that giving money to homeless people is the right thing to do either because it will prevent them from engaging in other activities such as crime, or because it will keep them from going hungry. In this line of argument, you are clearly thinking about the consequences (preventing a future crime, preventing someone from starving). Giving money based on such an argument would therefore fit within the consequentialist perspective. You may also believe that you should not help homeless people because they should be able to look after themselves, and that giving them money will only maintain their dependency on begging or even encourage them to use drugs or alcohol. Again, this line of argument, whether you agree with it or not, involves thinking about the consequences of doing one action or another.

However, simply looking at the consequences is not sufficient for making a decision. You need to decide which consequences are more important so that you can act in a particular way. An exploration of the consequences, therefore, may help to begin a process of reasoning, but it does not provide you with sufficient direction for making the right decision, or one that would be considered just. We therefore need to further our understanding of Utilitarianism in order to guide our action in a manner that is just.

Many forms of Utilitarian ethics were developed over the course of a 100 years. It includes the work of Francis Hutcheson (1694–1746), Jeremy Bentham (1748–1832) and John Stuart Mill (1806–1873). While all these philosophers developed their theories around the importance of consequences, in this section on Utilitarian ethics we will focus solely on Mill's version, although we acknowledge that some of the earlier forms of the theory have influenced the development of what is presented here.

Briefly, Utilitarian ethics, including Mill's, is often recognised as promoting 'the greatest good for the greatest number'. As Almond (1985: 7) explains, for a Utilitarian, 'a multiplicity of individual interests – what is good for each member of society – make up the common interest, what is good for all, or at least

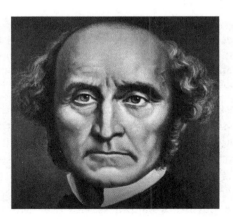

John Stuart Mill
Source: © Pictoral Press Ltd/Alamy

Did you know?

Before Mill shifted the focus of Utilitarianism to quality and quantity, his predecessor Jeremy Bentham thought that pain and pleasures could simply be measured quantitatively according to seven criteria:

- Intensity
- Duration
- Certainty
- Extent
- Remoteness
- Richness
- Purity.

The action that, according to these criteria, would produce the greatest amount of pleasure (in terms of quantity) would ensure the best outcome.

What do you think of this? What would be the main difficulties in applying this earlier version to social work?

the most'. In other words, according to Utilitarian ethics, the right action will be the one that maximises the welfare of the greatest number of people affected by it. Therefore, looking at the consequences, the right action will be the one that promotes the best outcome for the most people. To refine our understanding and to avoid oversimplifying this slogan so that it fits every situation, we will now examine the two concepts that make it up and define what Mill understood as constituting the 'greatest good' for the 'greatest number'.

The concept of 'greatest good'

The creed which accepts as the foundation of morals, utility, or the greatest happiness principle, holds that actions are right in proportion as they tend to promote happiness, wrong as they tend to produce the reverse of happiness. By happiness is intended pleasure, and the absence of pain; by unhappiness, pain, and the privation of pleasure (Mill 2004: 9–10).

To define the greatest good, Mill suggests that we look at the concepts of 'pain' and 'pleasure'. For Mill, the greatest good correlates with the outcome that will produce the most pleasure and the least pain. Indeed, Mill believes fundamentally that every man and woman always tries to maximise pleasure and minimise pain. While this may be debatable, Mill thought that the more people have pleasure, the happier they are likely to be. The pursuit of pleasure, therefore, corresponds with the pursuit of happiness. However, Mill warns us to consider not only the quantity, but also the quality of pain and pleasure that an action may procure. For example, a person may have many acquaintances (quantity) but have no real friends (quality). Is this person happier than someone who has one or two real friends? This shows the importance of both quality and quantity in the assessment of pain and pleasure. Therefore, building from the work of Jeremy Bentham, Mill believes that we must look at both the *quantity* and the *quality* of pleasure in a given situation. As Mill explains:

> According to the greatest happiness principle, the ultimate end, with reference to and for the sake of which all other things are desirable (whether we are considering our own good or that of other people), is an existence exempt as far as possible from pain, and as rich as possible in enjoyment both in the point of quantity and quality; the test of quality, and the rule for measuring it against quantity, being the preference felt by those, who in their opportunity of experience to which must be added their habit of self-consciousness and self-observation, are best furnished with the means of comparison (2004: 17).

Thus, the greatest good can be assessed by examining whether the consequences of an action will lead to happiness by providing pleasure, which can be measured both qualitatively and quantitatively. However, is happiness not a subjective expression of feeling? How do we make sure – pain and pleasure apart – that one action will lead to more happiness than another? Is happiness always related to experiencing a maximum of pleasure and a minimum of pain? Is someone who likes some form of pain (a masochist) necessarily unhappy? An athlete training for the Olympics must go through considerable pain to achieve the goal of a medal. Does this not somehow contradict 'pleasure equals happiness'?

According to Mill, the happiness that an action confers also needs to be assessed in terms of its *utility*. The greatest good, for Mill, is therefore the course of action that maximises the quantity and the quality of happiness by virtue of its usefulness in a given situation. In other words, for a course of action to be right, it must not only promote happiness, but must also be useful to those involved.

However, can a situation always promote happiness for all those involved? For example, if you work with a service user who currently lives in the community and requires a high level of care, and her daughter, the only natural carer, is exhausted and demands that her mother be placed in residential care against the wishes of her mother, what course of action will you support based on happiness and utility? This example demonstrates competing demands that often cannot be maximised simultaneously. Of course, you would undertake a thorough assessment of the situation and have in hand all the relevant policies and legislations, but the fundamental question remains: whose happiness should you favour? To assess the rightness or the wrongness of an action in terms of Utilitarian ethics, we must therefore not only look at the consequences, but also determine those consequences that will promote the greatest happiness by virtue of their utility for the greatest number. We will now look at the second part of the slogan, the 'greatest number', to further explore the concept of utility.

The concept of greatest number

Simply put, what is considered as promoting the greatest good, the greatest happiness, or as we have just seen, the greatest utility, is also what will produce an outcome benefiting the greatest number of people involved in a situation. This is supported by the belief that it is the sum of individual interests that makes up the collective interest. As Almond (1985: 7) explains, 'For a Utilitarian, a multiplicity of individual interests – what is good for each member of society – make up the common interest – what is good for all, or at least the most.' For the Utilitarian, then, the ethically right action is that which maximises the welfare of the greatest number of people based on utility. This, of course, requires that we take utility into consideration when conducting assessments because, as outlined in the example above, we may be in a situation that pits one person against the other (older person's needs vs. those of the carer). Vardy and Grosch (1999) provide an interesting example to illustrate this point in their discussion about Utilitarian ethics. They explain that abortion is neither good nor bad (because it involves one person against another); however, it only becomes a question of rightness or wrongness when we consider to what end the abortion is being performed, that is, how it satisfies the greatest good for the greatest number in terms of its utility. Therefore, the authors suggest that abortion is morally acceptable if it is used to control the birth of a tenth child in a low-income family but immoral if it is performed on a young married women because it interferes with her career (Vardy and Grosch 1999). The concept of utility and of the greatest number is clearly illustrated in this example.

Another important point in the Utilitarian theory of justice is that one's decision making should remain impartial. As Mill explains, 'All persons are deemed to have the right to equality of treatment except when some recognised social expediency requires the reverse' (Mill 2004: 93). This means that equal rights should be upheld as much as possible, unless some conditions that promote the greatest good for the greatest number require us to act otherwise. Therefore, according to the Utilitarian perspective, in order to act ethically you may have to compromise your own interests with those of others. In this sense, this theory views justice as balancing private interest with public interest.

The greatest good for the greatest number as a method of ethics

We have seen that the morally right action is defined in terms of its consequences with regard to the utility it brings in a given situation. As such, act-Utilitarianism will support an action as morally good as long as the action itself is conducive to general happiness. It is the value of the consequences of one act or another that is then used to examine general happiness. For example, a social worker in a food bank has just conducted an assessment and realises that the needs of the service user in question are valid but that the service user's particular situation does not meet the eligibility criteria. Applying the principle of the greatest good for the greatest number, as we have seen, would require examining the consequences of action or non-action in this situation in terms of its utility for the various parties.

The two basic actions that could be taken in this situation are as follows: the social worker bends the rules and offers food to the person, or the social worker does not bend the rules and does not offer food to the person. Applying the Utilitarian perspective would mean weighing the different consequences. Simply put, we could argue that bending the rules would result in the family having access to food, and since this only involves one family, the other service users may not feel the effect. On the other hand, not giving the food to the family may result in further problems for the family. Therefore, through the simple application of the greatest good for the greatest number, it would be justifiable to bend the rules because it would promote the happiness of most people in this situation, that is, the family. This way of applying the greatest good for the greatest number is called the act-Utilitarian perspective. Act-Utilitarianism, in its simplest form, is founded on the belief that 'every action should be taken so as to maximise happiness' (Graham 2004: 144). This means that you must consider the whole situation and weigh each consequence in terms of its utility for all those involved.

As you may have surmised from the above example, the act-Utilitarian perspective may present some problems in that it can be too permissive or be used to justify many actions, even unethical ones, if the value of a particular course of action in terms of its consequences can be considered above all others.

For example, as Mill explains in his book *Utilitarianism*:

> It appears from what has been said that justice is a name for certain moral requirements, which regarded collectively, stand higher in the scale of social utility and are therefore of more paramount obligation than any others; though particular cases may occur in which some other social duties are so important as to overrule any one of the general maxims of justice. Thus, to save a life, it may not only be allowable, but a duty, to steal or take by force the necessary food or medicine or kidnap and compel to officiate the only qualified medical practitioner (Mill 2004: 93–4).

What is the difference between act- and rule-Utilitarianism?

Act-Utilitarianism is based on the prediction of the consequence of one particular action. As long as the outcome will produce the greatest happiness for the greatest number, the action can be justified.

Rule-Utilitarianism is similar to the act version but claims that the action will only be good if the consequences are good and the action is universalisable into law.

In other words, act-Utilitarianism should be used with caution, and it is in this context that we will now look at a variation of this perspective: 'rule-Utilitarianism'.

Rule-Utilitarianism

Rule-Utilitarianism suggests that, instead of being determined by the utility of the difference/consequence of one particular action, our actions should be determined by *rules* that, if generally followed, would lead to the greatest happiness (Graham 2004). Such rules take priority over individual actions and do not allow for exceptions. Therefore, the greatest good for the greatest number still applies, but for a *rule* as opposed to a single situation. Indeed, under rule-Utilitarianism, rules are developed under Utilitarian principles, that is, they promote the greatest happiness for the greatest number: if followed, they will lead to morally right action; if not, they will lead to morally wrong action. Let us now return to the example of the social worker who must decide whether or not to bend the rules at a food bank for a particular service user. We saw that under act-Utilitarianism, bending the rules may be deemed morally right in such a situation. Let us now consider the same situation under the rule-Utilitarian perspective. We now must define a rule that will apply to everyone. We may ask if it is morally right to bend a rule if a service user needs a service that they cannot access otherwise. We must now determine whether this rule would lead to the greatest good for the greatest number for all similar cases. Obviously, if rules are bent to meet every exception, the system would soon fall apart. In this sense, the rule applied in this case would become useless and not produce the greatest good for the greatest number, and resources, which are always limited, would not be sufficient to help those who truly need them, that is, the majority of users. Therefore, under the rule-Utilitarian approach, bending the rule would not be morally right since it would not promote the greatest happiness for the greatest number. To achieve the greatest happiness, everyone must obey the rule, and for the principle to be Utilitarian, it must maximise utility for the greatest number.

Rule-Utilitarianism is useful in so far as that instead of simply weighing the consequences of one action, it looks at the rule that, if applied to a given action, would maximise the welfare of the majority. Rule-Utilitarianism may therefore help to counteract some of the difficulties associated with act-Utilitarianism.

The ultimate end of both versions of Utilitarian ethics is to serve the majority of people involved in a situation. Therefore, using both approaches in the resolution of an ethical dilemma may help in weighing right and wrong actions by examining the consequences they have on society in general. For the Utilitarian,

Justice is a name for certain moral requirements, which regarded collectively, stand higher in the scale of social utility, and are therefore of more paramount obligation

Reflection break

1 Try to summarise the two versions of Utilitarian ethics.

2 What are the main differences between act-Utilitarianism and rule-Utilitarianism?

3 How do you feel they can be applied to ethical deliberation in social work?

4 Can you see any limitations in applying them to social work practice?

5 How can these perspectives help you in dealing with ethical dilemmas related to social justice?

than any others; though particular cases may occur in which some other social duties is so important, as to overrule any one of the general maxims of justice (Mill 2004: 54).

We said at the beginning of the chapter that the rules of society are largely influenced by the Utilitarian tradition in that many laws are created to suit the majority, and thus achieve greatest utility for the greatest number. Anti-social behaviour orders are clearly an example of Utilitarian policies that are established so that the majority can live happily without a 'troubling minority'. In addition, various codes of conduct are influenced by Utilitarian values (Banks 2006, Rhodes 1986).

Although Utilitarianism ethics is considered one of the main approaches to ethics in social work (and one of the three moral perspectives we have chosen to cover in Part 3 of this book), a chapter on social justice would not be complete without discussing, even briefly, another theory of justice, that of John Rawls. Not only will this theory help us further our understanding of social justice, but it will also address some of the limitations identified above with regard to Utilitarian ethics.

Rawls's theory of justice

John Rawls (1921–2002), an American born in Baltimore, USA, was one of the most important political philosophers of the twentieth century. His theory of justice was inspired by many Kantian principles (see Chapter 6) and was developed as an attempt to oppose some of the premises articulated in the Utilitarian

Rawls (1971) on equality, fairness and justice

Rawls understands **equality** in terms of positions between people, whereas he discusses **fairness** in terms of procedures in deliberation. **Justice** is the result contained in the principles that have emerged as a process of equality and fairness in defining principles.

perspective. As such, the aim of his work was to establish fundamental principles that, if followed, would provide a model for organising social life based on cooperation and consensus.

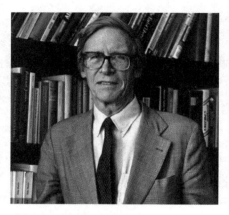

John Rawls
Source: Jane Reed/Harvard University News Office

He spent the greater part of his life working at Harvard University, where he published his *Theory of Justice* (1971). Rawls attempted to formulate principles of justice that, instead of favouring the majority (as in Utilitarianism), would consider each person as equally important and worthy. As such, Rawls proposed a conception of justice equated with fairness. Indeed, by defining a basis for equality and fundamental rights, his theory is an attempt to establish principles in which the rights of individuals are central, but also in which inequalities are impossible to avoid. Such a conception provides minimal protection for the oppressed and marginalised of society (Rawls 1971). Rawls's theory of justice also proposes a shift away from Utilitarian principles of ethics, in which justice is no longer understood as a matter of utility and majority of interests, but instead as a matter of fairness and fundamental liberties.

The conditions for a theory of justice: social contract, original position and the veil of ignorance

The basis of Rawls theory is what he calls a 'social contract'. For Rawls, a social contract involves a set of rules that, through reason, are determined and agreed upon by everyone in a given society. Once agreed, the social contract is to be maintained by the state and its political system,[1] which will then provide

---

[1] It must be noted that Rawls refers in his theory to liberal democratic political systems.

Rawls's social contract

A social contract is a form of agreement that people consent to live by in society.

What are the original position and the veil of ignorance?

Simply put, these two concepts provide the two necessary conditions for developing the principles of justice that will benefit people both individually and collectively.

The *original position* means that people are placed in a situation of equality, and the *veil of ignorance* implies that people develop the principles of justice without knowing what their condition would be in a hypothetical society; people therefore have no way of knowing how they would be personally affected by such principles.

the necessary conditions to ensure that people can achieve their goals and live a good life. A social contract in the Rawlsian sense involves basic liberties and equalities. Fundamental to this principle is the respect for individuals and their ability to reason, two concepts borrowed from Kant (see Chapter 6 for further discussion). The notion of social contact is fundamental to Rawls's theory of justice.

From this, a first question may be asked: how can we achieve Rawls's notion of social contract, that is, a contract that is determined and agreed by everyone? Indeed, how can self-interest be controlled in the definition of such a contract? Given that there are many power relationships in society, if a group is made up of individuals with different needs and interests, how can we guarantee that this group will be able to define and agree on rules that suit *everyone*? Can the interests of an unemployed single mother be represented on the same basis as those of a powerful banker? This represents quite a challenge, because a social contract is one that is *agreed upon by all individuals*. Rawls believes that this is possible as long as two conditions are met: the 'original position' and the 'veil of ignorance'. Let us now take a look at these two conditions.

The original position is a hypothetical situation in which everyone is placed in an *equal social position*. In the original position, there are no power relationships between the rich and the poor, or in terms of race, gender, sexuality, gender role, disability, culture, religion or any other difference that could generate social inequalities. Consequently, the original position requires people to forget about who they are and just 'be' as everyone else. However, given that such a situation is unlikely to occur (we live in a society with many social inequalities, and it is difficult to act against our own interests) Rawls adds a second condition – that people wear a veil of ignorance. Rawls explains that under the veil of ignorance, people 'do not know how the various alternatives will affect their own particular case, and they are obliged to evaluate the principles solely on the basis of general considerations' (Rawls 1971: 136). The veil of ignorance is a concept in which individuals must blindly decide on the rules that make up their social contract. In other words, under the veil of ignorance, that is, without knowing their future roles, status, position, cultural heritage, general health, religion, etc., people must define and agree on rules that are then used to organise social life. Thus, "If the individuals concerned do not know what position they will occupy in society, then it is rational for them to agree that each should receive a "fair distribution of primary social goods" (Fives 2008: 46). In other words, this process ensures that people from all walks of life have an equal representation in the definition of the principles of justice. Without an advantage in the original position and wearing the veil of ignorance, everyone should end up with the same principles as formulated by Rawls.

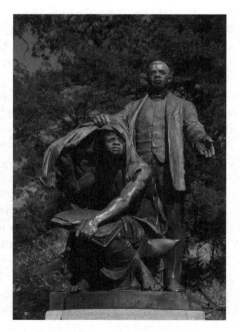

**Lifting the Veil of Ignorance –
Booker T. Washington Memorial**
Source: © The Protected Art Archive/Alamy

Reflection break

Imagine you are on a desert island with five other people. You are a recognised leader and have many strategic ideas. The other people are a pregnant woman, a child, a wounded doctor, a healthy man and a craftsman.

There is only enough food (one goat, two litres of milk, five litres of water and one kilogram of nuts) for three people to survive for one week until you find more resources.

1 Try to imagine how you would share the food. Define the principles you would use to share the food among yourselves. Take some notes about the reasons for your choices.

2 Now imagine you are in the original position and wearing the veil of ignorance. This implies that you are no longer the person who allocates the food and that you could be any of the people described above. Again, try to define some principles for sharing the food and note the reasons for defining such principles.

3 Are the principles you came up with the same as those when you were not in the original position and wearing the veil of ignorance?

Let us now explore the principles of justice as formulated by Rawls.

Rawls's principles of justice

You may have gathered in the reflection break that it is not any easy task to distribute limited resources or any other 'goods' in the Rawlsian sense. To achieve this task fairly, Rawls proposes two fundamental principles for allocating goods including liberties, opportunities and material goods:

1 The principle of equal liberty

2 The principle of equality of opportunity and the difference principle.

As you can see, these principles are numbered. According to Rawls, the order of these principles is important because only when the first principle (liberty) is met can the second principle be applied. There are also certain conditions under which this can happen. We shall now look at these principles in more detail.

Equal liberty

The first principle, related to basic liberties, reads as follows:

Each person has an equal claim to a fully adequate scheme of equal basic rights and liberties, which scheme is compatible with the same scheme for all; and in this scheme the equal political liberties, and only those liberties, are to be guaranteed their fair value' (Rawls 1993 in Lamont and Favor 2007: 5–6).

In other words, this principle tells us that all *basic liberties* must be equally distributed: what is allowed for one should also be allowed for all.

> **Rawls often refers to the concept of 'goods'. What does this concept mean in terms of the principles of justice?**
>
> For Rawls, the notion of goods to be distributed includes material goods, public services, wealth, power, etc. However, Rawls makes an important distinction between primary goods such as liberty of expression, political liberty, etc. and material goods such as wealth, financial resources, property, etc.

How, you may ask, can this be achieved? It is important to note that Rawls did not consider all types of goods to be of equal importance. Included in his first principle are only those goods related to fundamental rights, such as political liberty, liberty of expression and assembly, the freedom of personal property, that is, the liberty to think and to choose what one believes in. Other liberties such as having the right to own a big house or having a particular social status within a group or community are not covered by Rawls's first principle, which involves *basic fundamental liberties*. In defining what can be considered an acceptable social contract, Rawls comes to the conclusion that in the original position and under the veil of ignorance, individuals would likely accept this first principle as being fair. Indeed, if you had to define and agree on the principles of liberty but did not know what social position you would occupy in a future society or what religion you would practice (veil of ignorance), you would certainly agree on ensuring maximum rights and liberties.

Applied to social work, this principle may be interpreted as follows: regardless of age, gender, culture, class, ability, of any other aspect of people's lives that could be used to differentiate them from others, each person has the right to fundamental liberties. According to Rawls, this means that no matter who you provide services to, each person, by law, should be treated in the same way as others. Many of the fundamental liberties that Rawls cites can be found in such documents as the *Universal Declaration of Human Rights;* for example, Article 1: 'All human beings are born free and equal in dignity and rights.' You can see in this article that no attention is paid to a person's origin, age or any other distinctive feature. Clearly, in this principle, everyone is equal in terms of basic rights and liberties.

Now that the question of basic liberties is covered, you must wonder why there are so many inequalities in society. The first answer is that Rawls's principles are not necessary integrated or even interpreted everywhere the same way. Of course, while Rawlsian principles are recognised as extremely influential, how they are applied by each country may vary. For example, in the UK, some laws are still deemed incompatible with the *Universal Declaration of Human Rights*. You may recall the controversy around the detention of people under the Anti-Terrorism, Crime and Security Act 2001. Indeed, in the UK, the court has the right to make 'declarations of incompatibilities' between home legislations and the UN convention of human rights. The result, of course, is that not all of the human rights defined in the convention are applied in every country. Therefore, while Rawls's first principle is fundamental to many current UK acts and legislations, some of the liberties are not always compatible with regional legislation, and therefore, not everyone's access to these basic rights is guaranteed.

We shall now turn to the second principle of Rawls's theory of justice and examine how, where inequalities are unavoidable, society can still be based on social justice principles.

Equality of fair opportunity and the difference principle

How can we distribute equally goods that are not considered fundamental and that are scarce? What principle could we use to help us decide on the distribution of resources in the Reflection break exercise above?

Rawls proposes a second principle for achieving justice, but also reminds us that to apply this second principle we must ensure that the first principle has been satisfied. Rawls formulates his second principle as follows:

> Social and economic inequalities are to satisfy two conditions: (a) they are to be attached to positions and offices open to all under conditions of fair equality of opportunity; and (b), they are to be to the greatest benefit of the least advantaged members of society (Rawls 1993 in Lamont and Favor 2007: 5–6).

What Rawls is saying here is that if inequalities must exist in society they shall not be in regard to basic fundamental liberties, and they shall only be acceptable if they benefit the least advantaged of society. Let us explore what this means in practice.

Imagine a hypothetical situation in which a company wishes to recruit a new employee to perform a series of tasks that no one in the company is able or qualified to perform. The company decides to advertise the job at a higher salary than most employees receive because the job requires a higher qualification and involves many difficult tasks. According to Rawls, it may be acceptable to pay someone a higher salary, even though this could be considered 'unequal'. However, for it to be fair, you would need to satisfy two conditions: first, you would need to make sure that there are procedures that guarantee equal access to the job and that the opportunities for applying are fair. There are many levels at which this principle could be applied. First, there is the obvious equal opportunity strategy to be used in advertising the job, as well as a fair assessment of all candidate profiles. However, we could also apply the principle at a higher level and examine whether everyone of equal ability has the opportunity to develop their skills equally. Given the current social inequalities that exist in Britain, it is unlikely that such a situation would pass the first principle of justice as formulated by Rawls. Indeed, there are many inequalities with regard to access to education, for example. One could argue that not everyone of the same abilities has equal access to higher education, and therefore, this would not meet the first part of the second principle. Economic inequalities may prevent able people from accessing education. A just society, in Rawls's terms, would be one that promotes equal opportunity for equal ability, skills, etc. Therefore, if we return to our example above, even if the company puts various mechanisms in place to ensure equal opportunity in the hiring process, there would still remain other factors to consider regarding the second principle, that is, ensuring equal opportunity for everyone to meet the requirements of the job (e.g., ensuring higher education or overall life opportunities), but this would need to be analysed at a much higher level.

The second part of the principle explains that if inequalities are to be present in society, they must be for the benefit of the most disadvantaged of society. Therefore, to return to our example of a higher salary for a higher skilled job, according to Rawls, you could justify the higher salary only if it benefited everyone – both those who earn less in the company and society in general. However, how can this principle be achieved? Again, we would probably need to analyse the situation at a higher level and determine, for example, whether the higher salary means more tax revenues and whether these revenues are reinvested in social programmes to serve the most disadvantaged of society. While this example may be simplistic, it effectively demonstrates how the second principle can allow inequalities while still promoting a society based on fair principles.

Returning to our desert island exercise, you may begin to realise that Rawls's theory of justice is not quite suited to the management of routine ethical dilemmas but is more useful for defining and developing policies that are just. In fact, one of the critiques of Rawls's theory is that it is more a political philosophy than an ethical perspective. As such, while it helps us in understanding the concept of social justice in a certain way, it is more useful for examining the notion of justice and defining the principles of justice within institutions and organisations than it is for analysing ethical issues as in the Kantian and Utilitarian perspectives.

Having said this, applying Rawls's principles of justice to the desert island situation would require you to define principles for the distribution of the resources. Based on Rawls's principles, you could justify the decision of giving more food to those who are able to cross the island because it would give an advantage in the long term to those who are not able to. Indeed, those who are fitter to cross the island may need more resources to do so, but the inequality of the distribution of resources would be offset by the advantage it would bring to everyone. Therefore, what is considered a priori as unfair, that is, giving

Reflection break

1 Placing yourself in the conditions of the original position and the veil of ignorance, would you agree with the principles of justice as formulated by Rawls?

2 How would you apply these principles to the 'desert island' exercise above? How would you distribute the food?

3 What would be the difficulties of applying Rawls's theory of justice to the desert island example?

more food to a few, would be justified as fair according to Rawls, because such inequalities will eventually benefit the most vulnerable.

One critique of Rawls's theory is whether or not it is possible for individuals to fully detach themselves from their social and historical contexts when defining principles of justice. Indeed, the essence of the veil of ignorance is that individuals will make decisions not knowing where they are located in the socio-political spectrum of society. Another difficulty with Rawls's theory, which we will discuss in Chapter 8, is that for some moral theorists, it is neither possible nor desirable to distance yourself from your social and cultural and historical context when trying to understand ethical issues. Finally, some scholars argue that the concept of justice should not be analysed in terms of resources (or primary goods) but in terms of social practices (Mullaly 2010).

In sum, Rawls provides a useful framework for understanding the notion of social justice and proposes, through his theory, a way of achieving a society in which everyone agrees on the principles of justice. Rawlsian principles provide guidance not so much for practical action, such as managing an ethical dilemma in social work practice, but rather for orienting principles of justice with regard to policies or organisations.

In the first part of this chapter, we examined two different approaches used in philosophy and politics to understand the concept of social justice. We saw that Utilitarian ethics is commonly used in the welfare state and continues to influence some of the articles found in the codes of ethics of the UK and elsewhere. We also saw that Rawls's theory of justice helps to address some of the shortcomings of Utilitarian ethics, especially with regard to integrating some of Kant's principles (see Chapter 6). Nevertheless, both theories provide us with two valid frameworks for understanding and applying decisions in terms of justice. We now propose to look at a case study and to see how both the Utilitarian and the Rawlsian theories of justice can help us make decisions related to social work ethics.

Case study

Mourad's story

Mourad is a qualified social worker who works for the asylum seekers team in a Social Services Department of the West Midlands. He has been asked to assess Sithembiso, a young Zimbabwean woman who arrived unaccompanied after being picked up by the police two weeks ago at a service station in their Local Authority area. Since that time, she has been seeking asylum with the authorities.

Following a thorough psychosocial assessment in cooperation with other agencies, Mourad is of the opinion that Sithembiso is around 14–15 years old. However, the medical report states her age at over 16, most likely 17. When Mourad meets with his manager, Helen, to discuss the discrepancy between the team's report and the medical report, Helen takes the view that the medical report is most likely the correct one. When Mourad discusses the facts of the psychosocial assessment with Helen, she argues that Sithembiso is probably

(Continued)

claiming to be younger in order to benefit from the more generous support offered to unaccompanied asylum seekers under 16. She asserts that, based on the medical report, the official position of the department must be that Sithembeso is not entitled to any further support as an unaccompanied minor.

Mourad is concerned not only by this case, but also by a number of recent cases in which his team was convinced that the asylum seekers were under 16, even though the medical methods of age assessment, focusing mainly on dental X-rays, classified them as older. In addition, there is an emerging body of evidence that points to the questionable reliability of these tests for young people aged between 15 and 20 years and the inappropriateness of using such tests as the sole measure of age assessment. Mourad also feels that his manager's attitude reflects an increasing culture of cynicism and disbelief among the staff team. He has asked for a few weeks to be able to present evidence to the team concerning the problems of using dental records as the sole means of age assessment, but his request is repeatedly refused. Mourad's manager, Helen, has now asked him to modify his report and close the case.

Questions
Looking back through the case study:

1 Identify the ethical dilemma facing Mourad.

2 Identify the various courses of action Mourad can take.

3 Write down what you feel are the most important elements to consider in each course of action you identified above. Why do you feel these are important?

4 How would you express the issues facing Mourad in terms of social justice?

Analysis

The dilemma faced by Mourad raises many controversial issues. The main elements of the case are as follows:

1 Mourad is engaged in a professional relationship with Sithembiso;

2 Mourad estimates Sithembiso's age at less than 16 years;

3 The medical examination estimates her age at more than 16 years;

4 The manager and the department are of the opinion that the medical report is correct;

5 Mourad is aware that some dental X-rays are not reliable in estimating the age of service users between 15 and 20 years;

6 Mourad is in disagreement with the department position; and

7 Helen asks Mourad to modify his report.

We will now analyse the case study using the Utilitarian and the Rawlsian perspectives because these are good starting points for analysing cases involving issues related to social justice and the provision of services.

We believe that using these two theories will help our analysis at two different levels: the first, ethical issue, which we believe can be formulated as an ethical dilemma, is that Mourad is faced with the choice between continuing to support Sithembiso's claim that she is 15, or modifying his report as demanded by his manager; the second, broader ethical issue we observed in this case is related to social justice and inequalities within the Social Service Organisation, which are apparent in the views of the staff team and the agency.

Before analysing the ethical issues outlined above, we will look at various codes of ethics in order to explore how the documentation of professional bodies can help to assess this case with regard to the management of ethical issues and justice. While we do not believe that ethics should be understood as a simple application of codes of ethics and conduct, it is always important to situate a dilemma within the parameters of such codes. As such, these codes are a useful starting point, especially as a reminder of professional values. The table below lists some articles that we have found useful to the analysis of Mourad's story.

British Association of Social Workers Code of Ethics	General Social Care Council Code of Practice (2002, revised April 2010)
Responsibility for relieving and preventing hardship and for promoting wellbeing is not always fully discharged by direct service to individuals, families and groups. Social workers have a duty to:	1 As a social care worker, you must protect the rights and promote the interests of service users and carers.
Bring to the attention of those in power and the general public, and where appropriate challenge ways in which the policies or activities of government, organisations or society create or contribute to structural disadvantage, hardship and suffering, or militate against their relief;	1.3 Promoting equal opportunities for service users and carers; and
	2 As a social care worker, you must strive to establish and maintain the trust and confidence of service users and carers.
Use professional knowledge and experience to contribute to the development of social policy;	3 As a social care worker, you must promote the independence of service users while protecting them as far as possible from danger or harm.
	This includes:
Promote social fairness and the equitable distribution of resources within their work, aiming to minimise barriers and expand choice and potential for all service users, especially those who are disadvantaged, vulnerable or oppressed, or who have exceptional needs;	3.1 Promoting the independence of service users and assisting them to understand and exercise their rights;
	3.2 Using established processes and procedures to challenge and report dangerous, abusive, discriminatory or exploitative behaviour and practice;
Challenge the abuse of power for suppression and for excluding people from decisions which affect them;	3.3 Bringing to the attention of your employer or the appropriate authority resource or operational difficulties that might get in the way of the delivery of safe care;

▶

British Association of Social Workers Code of Ethics	General Social Care Council Code of Practice (2002, revised April 2010)
Support anti-oppressive and empowering policies and practices, and to aim to assist individuals, families, groups and communities in the pursuit and achievement of equitable access to social, economic and political resources and in attaining self-fulfilment, self-management and social well-being;	3.1 Informing your employer or an appropriate authority where the practice of colleagues may be unsafe or adversely affecting standards of care;
Service in the interests of human well-being and social justice is a primary objective of social work. Its fundamental goals are:	5.6 Condone any unlawful or unjustifiable discrimination by service users, carers or colleagues (GSCC 2002a).
• To meet personal and social needs;	
• To enable people to develop their potential;	
• To contribute to the creation of a fairer society (BASW 2002).	

We have thus identified, in both the GSCC and BASW codes, several articles that would support Mourad in his defence of Sithembiso. While our intention is not to provide a list of all the articles that apply in this case, we have identified some articles from both codes that we believe would be important and applicable to Mourad's situation. We would, however, invite you to do this exercise yourself to see which articles you feel are relevant to Mourad's case.

From a consequentialist perspective, a breach of Code of Ethics could lead to professional discipline of a worker. Indeed from a BASW perspective, members alleged to have committed professional misconduct – defined as a practice that is harmful to clients or members of the public, prejudicial to the development or standing of social work practice, or contrary to the Code of Ethics – may be referred to the disciplinary board (BASW 2002). From a GSCC perspective, registered social workers who fail to comply with the Code of Practice may be found in breach. In cases where misconduct is judged serious enough to question a registrant's suitability to remain on the register, the GSCC can remove, suspend, or deregister the registrant from social work (GSCC 2002a). For a social worker these are serious consequences, and we will take these into consideration in the analysis below.

A justice perspective according to Utilitarian ethics

In line with the Utilitarian perspective, the first step would be to identify the different consequences that would emerge as a result of the different courses of action. For the purposes of our analysis, we will focus on the following dilemma faced by Mourad, who has two options:

1 Maintain his position that Sithembiso is under 16 years of age;

2 Accept the manager's decision and modify his report accordingly.

We propose to use an adapted version of the grid developed by Legault (1999) to examine the possible consequences of both alternatives (referred to as A and B in the table) for all parties involved.

	Possible consequences if A		Possible consequences if B	
	Positive	Negative	Positive	Negative
Mourad	• Maintain a trusting relationship with Sithembiso • Act in the best interest of the service user • Act in accordance with both the code of ethics and the code of conduct: avoid possible professional disciplinary actions	• Bring trouble upon himself; challenging the manager could have negative repercussions on his work relationship with the manager and the agency	• Protect himself from difficulties with the manager and the agency	• Damaging the relationship with Sithembiso • May be in breach of code of ethics (BASW) and code of practice (GSCC) • May increase Sithembiso's level of distress
Sithembiso	• Have access to a package of services more adapted to her identified need • Maintain trust towards Mourad and the social work profession • Decrease anxiety • More likely to be continuously engaged in education; to become more socially integrated (Wade *et al.* 2005)	• None	• None	• Will only have access to a less appropriate level of care • May increasingly feel anxious • Damaged relationship with Mourad • Damage trusting relationship towards other social work professionals • Will lead to many complications with getting services

▶

	Possible consequences if A		Possible consequences if B	
	Positive	Negative	Positive	Negative
Manager	• Indirectly, may lead her to review the management style of the department and team	• May be perceived as a challenge to her authority and could have an effect on the staff team • Could be perceived indirectly as a challenge to social work services	• Maintain status quo	• Maintain status quo
Agency	• Indirectly, may lead to a review of policy and the broader organisational culture	• May be perceived as a challenge to management structure • May affect the budget of the agency and, indirectly, the distribution of other services	• Maintain status quo	• Maintain status quo • Maintain structure that promotes social injustice
Other service users/the broader environment	• May promote fairer access to services for a small number of service users, i.e. unaccompanied child asylum seekers	• May affect other service users with regard to resource allocation	• Maintain status quo • Maintain current level of resources for other services	• Maintain status quo • Continue to support a culture that does not promote fair access to services or equality of opportunity

The act-Utilitarian perspective

You will remember that act-Utilitarianism defines an action as morally good as long as the action itself is conducive to general happiness. We also asserted that it is the value of the consequences of one act or another that we then use to examine general happiness. Looking back at Mourad's case and both the positive and negative consequences emerging from the two possible courses of actions, we can now begin to apply the principles of the act-Utilitarian perspective.

As such, we will analyse the dilemma through the consequences in terms of general utility for the greatest number.

In examining the consequences above, it seems that one particular course of action may maximise happiness or utility for the greatest number, and therefore be considered a more ethical course of action according to the act-Utilitarian perspective. For example, if Mourad decides not to continue supporting Sithembiso in her claim that she is 15, despite having access to strong evidence in support of this claim, the most important consequence seems to be for Sithembiso, who would still have access to some resources, although not as extensive as those if she were assessed as 15 years old. Another important consequence is that Sithembiso may lose her trust in Mourad and in the social work profession. We know, indeed, that trust is an essential component of work with unaccompanied child asylum seekers (Kohli and Mitchell 2007). A consequence for Mourad is that he could be disciplined by one of the social work regulators or professional associations. However, for this to happen, a complaint would need to be filed, and looking at the case study, it is unlikely that this would be carried out by the agency, a colleague or even Sithembiso, who is in a vulnerable situation. Remember that according to Utilitarian principles, private interests need to be situated and weighed if they are to serve public interest; it is therefore unlikely, on this basis, that a disciplinary action towards Mourad from a regulator would be sufficient to justify a different course of action. On the other hand, discontinuing support for Sithembiso by modifying his report could be seen, at this time, as promoting the greatest utility for the greatest number, considering the consequences for the staff team, the agency and more indirectly, the population using all services.

Therefore, in this case, from an act-Utilitarian perspective, the right course of action, that is, the one seen as promoting the greatest utility for the greatest number, would be for Mourad to modify his report.

As we observed in the theoretical section above, act-Utilitarian ethics can be seen as sometimes justifying unacceptable behaviours. First of all, we must remember that deliberation here is based upon a series of predicted consequences. However, it is difficult to assess the extent to which our prediction will be correct, and therefore a simple application of act-Utilitarian perspective, as seen above, may still lead to a wrong action. This is mainly because

Reflection break

1 Think back on the criticism of the act-Utilitarian perspective. Do you feel that this perspective promotes the principles of social justice in this case? Why or why not?

2 Considering that many decisions are based on act-Utilitarian principles, how do you feel the understanding of this perspective influences your view of ethics?

act-Utilitarian only considers the present situation in its analysis. As we have shown in this example, the act-Utilitarian perspective can lead to wrong actions even if they may be justifiable theoretically. Therefore, while we do not believe that the analysis above constitutes the ethical way forward to manage the dilemma of this particular case study, we felt it was necessary to demonstrate this theory in action: understanding act-Utilitarianism and being able to apply its principles may help to see *ethically* more clearly. As in Francis Bacon's famous adage, 'knowledge is power'. It is therefore by understanding how principles that are still dominant in society can affect decision making that one can develop a platform for resisting them in practice. Let us now explore how the rule-Utilitarian perspective can inform decision making in this case.

The rule-Utilitarian perspective

As we noted earlier, rule-Utilitarianism addresses some of the criticism towards act-Utilitarianism by suggesting that our actions should not be determined by the consequences of the actions themselves, but instead by the rules that would bring the greatest happiness or utility. Applying the rule-Utilitarian perspective in Mourad's case means finding a rule that, if respected in all cases, would lead to the greatest utility. The question is: what sort of rule would help us achieve the right course of action according to this perspective?

We saw that, according to the act-Utilitarian perspective, Mourad may be inclined to modify his report to bring the greatest utility to the greatest number of people. Could we make a universal rule out of this possible course of action? In other words, could we define a rule that, if generally followed, would justify Mourad's action?

We saw above that values expressed in various codes of ethics would be in opposition to modifying the report. Could we then arrive at an ethical rule by saying that 'breaching a professional code of ethics is acceptable if it benefits the greatest number of people involved in a given situation'? Upon analysis, it would be difficult to universalise this rule because if codes of ethics can be broken, what is the point of having rules at all? We could argue that it would not be promoting the greatest good for the greatest number because such rules would be useless. Therefore, the rule-Utilitarian perspective in this case would not be in favour of Mourad breaching his professional codes of ethics because the consequences would be detrimental to the general population. Indeed, professional codes of ethics in social work or other disciplines are usually developed, among other things, to protect the population from misconduct. Therefore, according to a rule-Utilitarian perspective, it would be wrong to breach the professional code, and therefore this perspective would justify Mourad's continued support of Sithembiso's claim.

We will now examine a final theory to see what, in terms of justice, would be the right action in Mourad's case.

Rawls's theory of justice

As we noted at the beginning of this section, in addition to presenting an ethical dilemma, the case here indirectly raises broader issues related to social justice and inequalities, two dimensions that are apparent in the views of the staff team and the agency. In this sense, Rawls's theory of justice may be useful. Indeed, applying the original position and the veil of ignorance in this case may be helpful in underlining the beliefs that may be at the root of the situation. For example, it would be useful to consider whether the staff team, manager and agency would still maintain a culture of disbelief and cynicism regarding unaccompanied child asylum seekers children if they themselves had to define the principles of justice that apply in the case. The first principle, that of basic liberty for all, would certainly not be apparent in this case. Indeed, broadly speaking, this principle resonates with Article 2 of the United Nations *Declaration of Human Rights* (1948), which states:

> Everyone is entitled to all the rights and freedoms set forth in this Declaration, without distinction of any kind, such as race, colour, sex, language, religion, political or other opinion, national or social origin, property, birth or other status. Furthermore, no distinction shall be made on the basis of the political, jurisdictional, or international status of the country or territory to which a person belongs, whether it be independent, trust, non-self-governing or under any other limitation of sovereignty.

Accordingly, an asylum seeker, minor or not, should be treated the same way as a UK citizen or a permanent resident. However, we have already explained above that some human rights may be deemed incompatible with certain laws of this country.

Having said that, UK legislation requires that 'unaccompanied asylum seeking minors will have legal status under the Children Act 1989 and the Children (Leaving Care) Act 2000 in England and Wales and other primary and secondary child welfare statutes' (Simmonds and Merredew 2010: 1). This, however, may not be consistently applied country-wide because some councils may face problems due to limited resources and the associated costs. However, justice in terms of Rawlsian principles would mean that all councils treat every child equally, using the same rules, regardless of the child's origin or citizenship status. However, because the services are not organised in such a way as to achieve justice in a Rawlsian sense, Mourad would have to at least maintain and defend his position so that Sithembiso could have access to the services she needs. Indeed, whether Sithembiso is 15 or 17, under Rawls's first principle, she should have access to adequate placement. Mourad maintaining his position would at least guarantee this. Otherwise, Sithembiso would likely be placed in unsupported housing and experience the same difficulties that many unaccompanied minors who are not ready to live independently do (Wade *et al.* 2005). Rather, Sithembiso should be given access to a placement that provides security and opportunities for building new attachments

(Wade *et al.* 2005). Rawls's first principle of justice would also require Mourad to take the necessary actions to challenge the culture that exists in his organisation so that all unaccompanied minor asylum seekers are treated the same way as UK children in need of care.[2]

Because Rawls's first principle is not met – and, as we have stressed, only when the first principle is met can the second principle be applied – we cannot proceed with the application of the second principle. Indeed, only when basic liberties are applied equally can inequalities be tolerated and utilised in order to benefit the less advantaged. Clearly, in this case study, this first principle is not satisfied. Unaccompanied child asylum seekers are among the most vulnerable in society and are disadvantaged by many policies – from age assessment to detention. In addition, as Simmonds and Merredew explain,

> They [child asylum seeker] will encounter negative portrayals of asylum seekers in the media, racism and stereotyping in their daily lives. There is a risk that their asylum claim will be refused and they will be returned to their country of origin. This may for some include detention as these issues are worked through (2010: 2).

The situation presented in this case study and relative to unaccompanied child asylum seekers in the UK generally may be qualified as unjust and therefore unethical according to both Rawlsian and rule-Utilitarian principles. Fortunately, the situation facing unaccompanied minor asylum seekers may change in the near future because the High Court recently ruled that, under the Children Act 2004, the Local Authority has the responsibility for ensuring that accommodation is available where the welfare of the young person requires it. Local authorities will therefore have to provide accommodation for 18-year-old asylum seekers leaving care (Griffiths 2010). Either way, the two theories of justice examined in this chapter will provide you with a framework for assessing various issues related to child asylum seekers or to other dilemmas in social work practice that involve questions of social justice or equality.

Summary

We have seen that both Mill's Utilitarian ethics and Rawls's theory of justice propose principles that can be applied to practical situations and help us analyse ethical issues and dilemmas related to social justice and equality. While these theories may be incompatible with one another, they provide two perspectives for analysing issues that are faced in practice. We have seen that Utilitarian ethics, as formulated by Mill, provides an understanding of justice that is oriented towards the concept of utility, and that a solution will be considered as long as it benefits the greatest number of people. We have

---

[2] This may involve contacting his professional association for support in this process.

emphasised that utility, which can be explored through an action's conse-quence, must be assessed both qualitatively and quantitatively. Rawls, on the other hand, proposes an understanding of justice involving an equally shared set of liberties and allowing for inequalities, as long as these inequalities ben-efit the less advantaged. Compared with other theories presented in this book, both theories provide us with further tools for understanding and managing the many complexities of social work practice in a variety of settings and involving populations facing numerous difficulties.

Further reading

If you are looking for complementary texts on application of Utilitarian perspec-tives to contemporary social problems, then we suggest you read Feldman, D. B. (2006) 'Can Suicide Be Ethical? A Utilitarian Perspective on the Appropriateness of Choosing to Die'. *Death Studies* 30 (6). This interesting text examines the question of suicide using Utilitarian principles. Feldman develops an argument to assert the wrongness or the rightness of suicide based on an analysis of consequences.

Also, you may find Smith Barusch, A. (2009) *Foundation of Social Policy: Social Justice in Human Perspective,* 3rd edn. Brooke/Cole, Belmont of interest. Written from a social policy and social work perspective, it explores the concept of justice. Although written for an American audience, it nevertheless manages to explore the concept of justice from a broad perspective, reviewing some of the concepts covered in our chapter and furthering the discussion. It also clearly demonstrates its application to social work practice.

CHAPTER 8

Professionalism in social work: character- and relationship-based approaches to ethics

In this chapter we will:

- Explore the notion of 'professionalism in social work' through character-and relationship-based ethical theory
- Present the theoretical foundations of Virtue Ethics and the ethics of care
- Illustrate how Virtue Ethics and ethics of care can be used to analyse an ethical dilemma in practice
- Discuss the strengths and weaknesses of the approach

Introduction

The two previous chapters discussed on the notions of self-determination, human dignity and social justice, which have been recognised as important key values in social work practice. The last concept we want to explore in this book is that of 'professionalism', a term often found in many codes of conducts and ethics. To do so, Virtue Ethics and the ethics of care or the so-called 'relationship-based perspectives' are two pertinent ethical frameworks because they often refer to personal qualities which make up the professional conduct, such as integrity and competence, which social workers are expected to embody in their work with the various stakeholders, including service users, groups, organisations, communities and the state. It is therefore through this theme that we will examine this third broad perspective in moral philosophy, one that enables the contextualisation of the concept of personal qualities and stresses the importance of relationships.

Character- and relationship-based ethics

We have already introduced the difference between principle-based and character-based ethics earlier in the book (see section on ethics in Chapter 2 for further discussion), so we will not enter into a detailed discussion about this here. However, you may remember that the general terms character-based ethics and relationship-based ethics are usually related to the persons facing the ethical dilemma as opposed to a set of principles used to deliberate and guide their actions. Indeed, we saw in Chapters 6 and 7 how both Utilitarian and Kantian ethics are based on the application of a *set of principles* (universality for Kant, and every action should be taken so as to maximise happiness for some Utilitarians). On the other hand, character- and relationship-based ethical theories generally refer to a variety of notions such as Virtue Ethics and the ethics of care, which do not rely on principles to guide the action but instead on the type of person a social worker should be and on the type of relationship a social worker should develop with service users. In this case, the ethically good action will not be based on such or such principles to apply, but instead on the type of person the social worker should aim to become. Thus, as opposed to principle-based ethics discussed in previous chapters, Virtue Ethics and the ethics of care do not try to prescribe the principles to follow and consequently the types of behaviour that could be considered right or wrong, but instead establish what is considered to be essential qualities of the person facing the dilemma and the context in which action or social work intervention takes place.

To illustrate this, let us return to an example already discussed in Chapter 6. Imagine you are about to leave the office at 5 p.m. when one of the service users you already work with arrives at the office appearing very distressed. Your manager asks you if you would stay a little longer to deal with the situation. You know that this situation will probably keep you at the office much longer than what you had anticipated. However, you decide to stay and see the service user. Now, try to imagine the reason behind your decision. First, you could say that you are staying later because there is a person in distress and according to your profession and your work setting you have the duty to help this person and provide them with a service. Alternatively, you could say that you are staying to see that person simply because you are someone who is caring, professional and committed to your profession and therefore you see this person because you do not feel there is any other way of doing it. The former way of making the decision emphasises a principle you are following, duty of care and helping people in distress is part of your role within the agency, whereas the second reason for staying is justified by the sort of person you are.

We shall now consider in more detail two ethical traditions related to character-based ethics, and explore some of their similarities and differences before examining a case study. We will therefore draw a broad picture of what

Virtue Ethics and the ethics of care are and explore how these traditions can potentially help social workers to be more ethical in their work.

Virtue Ethics

Virtue Ethics originally derived from the works of Plato and Aristotle, two philosophers of ancient Greece who lived four centuries before Christ. Virtue Ethics is a form of moral perspective, much like Kantian and Utilitarian ethics, but emphasising the *type of person* needed for an ethical community to develop. For a life to be ethical, an individual's actions follow from the virtuous character traits that they have developed through the course of their life. Therefore, a person who strives to live an ethical life will aim at acquiring a set of positive character traits, or personal qualities which help them to behave morally well at any given time. We shall return to the notions of the good life and positive character traits later in this chapter.

Virtue Ethics was a popular approach until the development of other perspectives, such as Kantian and Utilitarian ethics, during the Enlightenment period. However, it regained popularity from the second half of the twentieth century. This return to Virtue Ethics was driven by philosophers who had a reaction against modern moral philosophy, such as Kantian and Utilitarian ethics, which for them were no longer adequate for understanding right from wrong. On this, MacIntyre (1985: 236), an influential philosopher in Virtue Ethics, asserts that the main problem with ethical perspectives that use principles to decide right from wrong is that often, the principles get themselves into conflicts. For example, what would you do in an ethical dilemma where the principle of 'respect for the person' (Kantian ethics) gets into conflict with the principle of 'utility' (Utilitarian ethics)? Indeed, for MacIntyre (1985), the central problem lies in the question 'How do we know which rules (or principle) to follow?'

Let us examine a simple situation involving a young offender who is repeatedly arrested by the police for doing graffiti on walls in the park and causing damage to other people's property. We have chosen this example precisely because graffiti is something that some people see as a form of social expression, while others see it as anti-social and causing criminal damage. From a Utilitarian perspective (see Chapter 7), the ethically right principle would be to

Did you know?

Virtue Ethics was the main way of discriminating between good and bad until the eighteenth century, but it decreased in popularity with the emergence of modern moral theories such as Kantian and Utilitarian theories. However, Virtue Ethics has started to regain popularity in philosophy and in social work since the early 1980s.

promote the greatest good for the greatest number and, therefore, to take the necessary steps to prevent the young person from visiting the areas where they are carrying out the graffiti through an Anti-Social Behaviour Order.

However, the young person, as an individual, deserves respect and should get the support he needs from his family, but will not be able to if an Anti-Social Behaviour Order is issued against him. This would go against the principles of the Kantian approach (see Chapter 6). Therefore, in such a situation, which principles should receive priority? While you may have your own opinion as to which course of action should be taken, we must acknowledge that both of these principles could be applied. Unfortunately, many situations like this involve conflicts of principles from different families of perspectives, such as those opposing autonomy with the greater good. This is where Virtue Ethics can help social workers reposition themselves in terms of ethical practice, because it does not rely on principles to apply to a certain situation, but instead is based on the sort of person who would act ethically.

The 'good life' from the perspective of Virtue Ethics

True goodness, according to what we have discussed above, relies not so much on which principles to apply in one situation or another, but on what sort of person one ought to be. Virtue Ethics, therefore, focuses on the character of a person because, according to this perspective, such personality traits will, generally speaking, have an impact on that person and on others in terms of who they are and what they do. For example, an empathic social worker will not display empathy because there is expectation of that quality in her work but because it is a quality that she has which transcends all of her behaviours.

But how do we know who is the right type of person that produces 'good' in society? This is where Aristotle draws from the concept of *eudemonia*, or supreme good, which is achievable through the finding of happiness. Virtue ethicists talk about the means to an end and the end in itself. Eudemonia is the ultimate end, and all humans strive to achieve it.

To define the ethical life, the virtue ethicist will therefore focus on examining what kind of person someone should be in order to achieve eudemonia. In this sense, a good person would exhibit good qualities, and this would have an effect on the good life in general and on the pursuit of happiness for both

Eudemonia

Aristotle believed that *eudemonia* was the ultimate purpose in life. Eudemonia is the ultimate good, which can be achieved through the pursuit of happiness (well-being). Eudemonia also promotes 'human flourishing' (Graham 2004).

one's self and for others. The definition of what constitutes the good life can be found in the concept of virtue.

Virtues

For the virtue ethicist, eudemonia, or the absolute good, can be achieved through the nurturing and cultivating of virtues. 'A virtue is not an unthinking habit, but rather involves an intelligent judgement about the appropriate response to the situation you are in' (Warburton 1999: 55). A virtue is therefore a personal quality that you develop over time which will help yourself and others to grow and be happy. In this sense, a virtue is a fine balance between too much and not enough of something. A virtue is a trait or character that has developed to a point of perfection. In this sense, Aristotle (1999), in his book *Nicomachean Ethics*, explains that because a virtue is perfection, people who display this virtue will always produce the perfect result by performing the right action in a given situation. A virtuous practice in social work, therefore, consists in the social worker cultivating and developing the character traits or personal qualities that will lead to the ultimate purpose – eudemonia – or in social work terms, a sort of *best ethical practice.*

Table 8.1 gives some examples of virtues and the relationship between their excess and lack thereof.

McBeath and Webb (2002) point out in relation to Virtue Ethics that Socrates differentiates between two types of virtues: intellectual virtues and moral

What is a virtue?

From the Greek word 'aretè' (excellence of character), a virtue is a human quality that is displayed appropriately through the use of practical reason in various situations, with the aim of promoting the well-being of people in general.
A virtue is a quality that is situated between having too much and not having enough of something.

Table 8.1 Some virtues and the relationship between their lack and excess

Lack of	Virtue	Excess
Indifference	Compassion	Excessive concern
Intemperance	Self-control	Self-denial
Vanity	Humility	Timidity
Cowardice	Courage	Recklessness
Dishonesty	Trustworthiness	Blind trust
Intolerance	Patience	Resignation

virtues. Moral virtues include character traits such as liberality and temperance and provide people with opportunities to examine their experience, whereas intellectual virtues are acquired by instruction and include character traits such as wisdom and understanding. Criticality is another example of intellectual virtue.

Aristotle tells us that a virtuous person will display many virtues at the same time. It is therefore only through a combination of a number of virtues that a person can be considered virtuous: exhibiting only one virtue would not be sufficient. Therefore, virtues come in sets; one cannot possess a single virtue without possessing others. To illustrate this point, let us examine some virtues that cannot exist without others: a *courageous* person will also be *temperate* because without *temperance*, a person would risk becoming reckless; a social worker who is *compassionate* will also be patient because being *compassionate* involves a desire to fully understand the suffering of others, which requires time and patience.

A person who develops a set of virtues (excellence of character) will therefore aim at reaching perfection in many aspects of their lives. Thus, a virtuous social worker will aim at developing and nurturing these qualities, even though such qualities may never be fully developed. The end result is eudemonia, whereas attempting to develop them is a means to an end. For example, the *wise* social worker is a person who uses their judgement, sensibility and comprehension in any given situation. According to the virtue ethicist, this type of person would promote eudemonia in general, their actions will be based not so much on plain application of principles but because they display the character traits needed to excel in her practice. An example of promoting eudemonia in social work practice in Britain would be the development of a type of practice that reflects the principles established by the International Federation of social workers, that is, a practice that respects the dignity of all humans and is based on the principles of social justice.

We understand, therefore, that a virtue is a personal quality that is developed and displayed in various situations. We now turn to the virtues that are required in social work and to the conditions for their development.

Practical reasoning

For the virtue theorist, virtuous character can be developed through reasoning. It is through habituation in reasoning that a person can develop virtues or positive character traits such as courage, justice and temperance. MacIntyre (1999) points to the development of reasoning abilities in people to unlock and cultivate virtues that are appropriate to practice, in this case, social work. The process of reasoning can help people make decisions and decide to perform good actions, and it is through reasoning at all times that people can

Practical reason

Practical reason, in terms of Virtue Ethics, involves both reflection and self-knowledge. It is an 'enquiry that provides us with grounds for the criticism, revision, or even rejection of many of our judgements, our standards of judgement, our relationships, and our institutions' (MacIntyre 1999: 157).

become virtuous. Morse (1999) asserts that only then will a virtuous person perform virtuous acts in any given moral situation.

To illustrate this point, let us now consider a social worker who is asked to comply with a policy that is promoted within the organisation for which she works, but that has the potential of compromising the social work value base. For example, the manager may ask her to reduce the size of a service user's care package, purely for financial reasons. The social worker may decide to implement the policy or not. Through reasoning, the social worker will have to think through the situation in context and consider carefully the different aspects emerging from the situation. The reasoning process, according to the virtue ethicist, will make the social worker adept at working out what is most appropriate in the situation. Let us imagine that the social worker decides that she cannot reduce the care package because it compromises the social work value base. Let us also say that the manager and his boss are both in disagreement with the social worker and insist that the social worker reduces it. If the social worker still thinks the action goes against the social work value base, and she carefully reasoned about every aspect, she may decide not to implement the policy. On the one hand, just doing what you are asked to do would not be virtuous because it means you lack courage. On the other hand, simply refusing to do something without the support of your colleagues may not necessarily be an act of courage, but one of recklessness or intemperance. The virtuous behaviour in this case would be to reason about the situation, to be wise and consider all possible avenues, and to be courageous enough to carry out the decision without lacking judgement. It may also involve a certain amount of patience from the social worker. A virtuous social worker may therefore decide to gain some time, to pursue the challenge to the policy by exploring different avenues, such as seeking support from a professional association. What is important to remember is that in Virtue Ethics the appropriate behaviour depends on who you are, what the context of the situation is and your ability to reason while making a decision. Only then can you draw from your intellectual virtues in order to decide what is good or bad, and reason as to the best course of action in a particular situation.

If we examine what essentially constitutes a virtue, it becomes clear that practical reasoning can help social workers better define their social work values. As MacIntyre points out, a virtue can be developed through strength of character. He explains that virtue is 'an acquired human quality' (1985: 191) rather than a feeling about rightness or wrongness. These personal qualities or 'virtues' have to be practised in order to become part of one's life, as opposed to a one-off 'act of heroism' (Lynch and Lynch 2006).

To give a practical example of how virtues can be developed, let us explore an ancient virtue praised in the early Greek community. Although 'physical strength' has nothing to do with social work practice today, we nevertheless believe that thinking about this virtue will help you grasp how other virtues, whether moral or intellectual, can be developed and nurtured. Why was physical strength a virtue in ancient Greece? Before the polis was developed, many small communities were living far apart from one another. Therefore, they could not rely on fast protection as people do with the modern police force or the army. In order to protect their community and village, people had to develop a certain physical strength to defend themselves. In this context, physical strength was considered an important virtue to protect the community and do good. Now, imagine that you have to develop this virtue. What do you need to develop physical strength? You will probably need to train regularly, work very hard and this will not happen overnight. It will also take more than one session at the gym. It may take months or even years before you become strong. As you may realise, developing physical strength will happen over time, with a lots of practice and dedication because to achieve excellence, you will have to pursue that training, even when things are difficult. If you stop training, you will also lose your physical strength. The same principle applies to developing other kinds of virtues. Whether we are talking about patience, trustworthiness or humility or criticality, these virtues or personal qualities will not develop overnight. Therefore, to develop patience for example, you will have to be exposed to many situations whereby your patience will be tested. It is through being exposed to these situations, and by reasoning on the way your feelings make you behave, that you may develop your patience even further.

Social work virtues

While Virtue Ethics as applied to contemporary social work practice has gained in popularity during the last few decades (McBeath and Webb 2002, Banks 2006, Clark 2005, Banks and Gallagher 2009), there is no formal, exhaustive list of which virtues are most suited to social work practice. However, it is through the ability to reason that social workers are in a position to identify which set of virtues are appropriate for the context of practice and to develop and nurture these virtues through their experience of working with service users.

Some virtues related to social work, such as temperance, magnanimity, gentleness, truthfulness, wittiness, friendliness, modesty and justice, have been identified by Lynch and Lynch (2006), as well as by Clark (2006). Banks and

Gallagher (2009) also point to another set of virtues appropriate to the fields of health and social care and thus useful in a social work framework: professional wisdom, respectfulness, care, trustworthiness, justice, courage and integrity. As we can see, therefore, there is no 'official list' of virtues consensually accepted by the social work community as social work virtues. This can actually be seen as a critique of Virtue Ethics, as articulated by Houston (2003: 819), who asserts that 'insufficient attention is given to the problem of how virtue is defined and established in the first instance'. While the topic of Virtue Ethics is still in the developmental stages, it is essential to remember that the notion of reason is indispensable in Virtue Ethics because it enables the social worker to explore and identify which set of virtues is important to achieve eudemonia in a given social work context. The social worker will then have to develop and nurture these virtues. We can now begin to understand the rationale behind the use of reasoning in determining what constitutes a virtue or set of virtues. The centrality of using reason needs to govern the practice and should not be considered merely a theoretical option. On this, Aristotle reminds us that a set of virtues is a voluntary acquired disposition which is defined under the guidance of a thoughtful person (Aristotle 1999).

From Virtue Ethics to the ethics of care

We have seen that the focus of Virtue Ethics lies in the development of an individual's excellence of character and in the pursuit of happiness through the use of practical reason. Another critique of Virtue Ethics, however, is that most virtue theories have been developed and furthered by men, and that 'feminine' traits of personality have been all but ignored (Banks 2006). As we saw above, Virtue Ethics is related to practical reason and does not emphasise the role of emotions, which are more the realm of women than they are of men. As Jaggar (2000: 348) confirms, 'throughout the history of Western ethics, the moral status of women has been a persistent though rarely central to the topic of debate'. It thus becomes clear that Virtue Ethics could be enhanced by taking into consideration a more feminine mode of ethical deliberation, which is the main thrust of this section on the ethics of care. Indeed, given that one of the views of Virtue Ethics is that it can complement other types of ethics

What is ethics of care?

Ethics of care, as developed by feminists such as Gilligan and Noddings, argues that 'traditional ethical perspectives such as Kantian, Utilitarian and Virtue Ethics lack the values and qualities that are usually associated with women, for example, caring and responsibility'.

(Banks and Gallagher (2009), we now propose to examine another character-based ethical theory that we believe can be successfully combined with Virtue Ethics to render the latter more compatible with feminine character traits.

Essential features of ethics of care

Ethics of care was born out of a critique of Kolhberg's stages of moral development, which according to Gilligan, are not entirely adaptable to women. Indeed, based on a critique of Kolhberg's methodology and her own research with women, Gilligan came to the conclusion that there were fundamental differences in the way men and women morally deliberate and as such, Kohlberg's stages of moral development are not universally applicable. Such criticism is still relevant today, and the point here is not to say that men reason in one way and that women reason in another. However, we want to stress that there are many times that a person may not feel comfortable applying a particular moral theory to their life precisely because such a theory does not account for relationships with others, which are central to the context in which a decision is made. For example, in terms of Virtue Ethics, justice may be an important virtue (always give others their due), but this may not be so simple to apply in practice. A person may be confronted with a situation in which they must decide between what is right for their family and what is right for someone else's family and may very well decide in favour of their own family. But can we affirm that such a person is acting unethically or without virtue? Is it not because of their relationship with their family? This is where the ethics of care can contribute significantly to social work.

In this book, we shall use the foundation of the ethics of care as an approach in ethics that emphasises the importance of relationships, responsibility and caring in its definition of ethical behaviour. Indeed, we understand social work as involving 'people in relationships of commitment to each other's well-being, often sanctioned by the state' (Dominelli 2009: 7). We therefore believe that the concept of relationships between people is an essential feature of social work practice and requires a type of ethics that can account for it.

Thus, an ethics of care based on this understanding is one that emphasises the importance not only of character (as in Virtue Ethics), but also of the

What are Kolhberg's stages of moral development?

Kolhberg defined six universal stages of moral development, which, according to his research, are applicable to everyone. These involve three different levels, from 'obedience and punishment' to 'application of ethical principles', the latter being the highest level of moral development. According to Kolhberg, not everyone progresses to the highest level.

relationships in which the ethical issues takes place and the centrality of such concepts as responsibility and caring in the definition of the morally right action. As such, the ethics of care emphasizes the roles of *mutual interdependence and emotional response,* as noted by Beauchamp and Childress (2001: 373):

> many human relationships involve persons who are vulnerable, dependent, ill, and frail . . . [and] the desirable moral response is attached attentiveness to needs, not detached respect for rights . . . The person who acts from rule-governed obligations without appropriately aligned feelings such as worry when a friend suffers seems to have a moral deficiency. In addition . . . insight into the needs of others and considerate alertness to their circumstances often come from the emotions more than reason.

Consequently, while Virtue Ethics does not emphasise the importance of emotion in defining virtues and deciding on the morally good action, the ethics of care emphasises that emotions can have a cognitive role and allow us to deal with situations that are not immediately resolvable using practical reasoning alone.

During the last decade, there has been increasing debate about the resemblances between Virtue Ethics and the ethics of care. For example, Halwani (2003) asserts that ethics of care should be subsumed under Virtue Ethics by constructing care as an important virtue, while Hugman (2005: 71) states that the ethics of care is more a framework for understanding ethics within concrete experiences of relationships than it is a 'grand moral theory'.

The rest of this chapter will thus be devoted to combining our understanding of Virtue Ethics with that of the ethics of care, with particular attention to the context of practice and the relationship between the social worker and the service user, an approach which we feel is promising. Let us now examine a case study to which we will apply both the perspectives of Virtue Ethics and the ethics of care. As such, we will explore the case study by considering 'care' as one of many virtues relevant to social work practice, paying particular attention to the relationship between the social worker and the service user. Although Virtue Ethics and the ethics of care may not be considered part of the larger family of principle-based approaches, we will nevertheless examine their application in light of the various codes of ethics and practice of social work. In this regard, we will not consider these codes as principles to follow

Reflection break

Thinking back on what you have just read about Virtue Ethics and the ethics of care:

1 Summarise what you consider to be the main point of virtue of ethics theory.

2 Summarise what you consider to be the main point of the ethics of care.

3 How might these principles be used in social work practice?

in the Kantian or Utilitarian sense, but instead as a reminder of a set of values that can help us develop the virtues that are relevant to our profession. We will then conclude this chapter by discussing the compatibility of this approach with practice in Britain.

Summary: Virtue Ethics and the ethics of care

Virtue Ethics and the ethics of care both stress the importance of the character of the social worker and the nature of the relationship in which the intervention or ethical dilemma takes place. Virtue Ethics emphasises that it is through practical reasoning and the nurturing of appropriate virtues or character traits that a person will promote eudemonia or perfect happiness. The ethics of care complements Virtue Ethics because it asserts that it is the nature of the relationship that determines what type of person one ought to be.

Case study

Ruth's story

Ruth is a 45-year-old white British social worker who works with a disability team in Scotland. She has two daughters, one who lives abroad, and another, with cerebral palsy, who lives nearby in a housing resource provided by another disability team. Ruth's experience as a mother of a child with a long-term illness and physical disability is what motivated her, in her late thirties, to study social work and obtain her qualification in order to help other families in similar situations.

Samantha is a 19-year-old white British woman living in a council estate near Glasgow. She accesses a number of services through her local learning disability team. Ruth is her social worker and case manager and has been working with Samantha since she moved to adult care 18 months ago. Samantha was born with Down syndrome and is currently waiting for the result of an assessment for autism. She has mild to moderate learning disabilities. Samantha attends a special school three days a week and a mainstream community college the rest of the week. The teachers at her mainstream school say that she is integrating well overall. She lives semi-independently in a small block of self-contained flats that include a bedroom, bathroom and kitchen. The block also includes an on-site support worker who provides ad hoc support to all residents, as well as a warden. Even though Samantha is very different from Ruth's daughter, Ruth sometimes feels that Samantha reminds her of her daughter, and this somehow affects her relationship with her. Last month, Samantha, who is a keen chat room user, told Ruth that she has met a man through Facebook. During the last three meetings of the disability team, Samantha has told Ruth that her new boyfriend plans to come and visit her at the weekend. By the way she describes him, it would appear that the man is considerably older than her. Samantha says that she is in love, and that deep down in her heart, she feels he is the one. Ruth, who wants to support Samantha appropriately, uses the opportunity to discuss notions of sexuality and respect of self and others. At the following meeting, Ruth notices that Samantha is not as dynamic as usual. When asked about the weekend, Samantha changes topic. A few weeks later, Ruth notices that Samantha has a bruise on her arm. When asked about it, Samantha appears shy and does not know what to say. However, the bruise appears to have been caused by someone grabbing her arm because of the appearance of finger marks. When Ruth asks Samantha about her relationship with her boyfriend, Samantha says that he sometimes gets 'stressed' while with her, but she prefers not to say anything because he said he would leave her, and deep down she is in love with him. Ruth is beginning to feel concerned about the situation. When the warden of the block calls Ruth's supervisor to report that a man has been visiting Samantha regularly for three weeks, Ruth is asked to take appropriate measures to end Samantha's relationship with her boyfriend.

Questions

Looking back through the case study:

1 Identify the ethical dilemma facing Ruth.

2 Identify the conflicting values and the various courses of action Ruth might take.

3 Write down what you feel are the most important elements to take into consideration in each course of action you identified above. Why do you feel they are important?

4 How would you express the issues facing Ruth in terms of Virtue Ethics and the ethics of care?

Analysis

The dilemma facing Ruth underlines many aspects of social work practice that relate to professionalism. Central to the case are elements that relate to setting appropriate boundaries and positioning oneself correctly between protecting and supporting the service user. Issues of confidentiality and respect for the person are also present in the case.

We now propose to examine how different virtues help shed light on the definition of an ethically good action. We will also observe how the role of emotions and the nature of the professional relationship can shape ethical practice. We will do this by examining some of the relevant virtues proposed by Banks and Gallagher (2009) and McBeath and Webb (2002), and how they impact on our comprehension of Ruth's story and the notion of professionalism overall. In particular, we will explore how the virtues of respectfulness, care, trustworthiness, justice, courage, integrity and criticality can help social workers become better professionals in their practice and maintain the social work value base.

Respectfulness

Respectfulness, in its simplest form, is showing respect for another person. For a social worker, this would mean respecting the values and views of the service user, even if these differ from one's own beliefs or personal experiences of similar situations. This means that Ruth would respect Samantha's desire to share (or not) her story with her and to continue seeing (or not) her boyfriend. In the case presented above, Samantha is deemed autonomous: she is living independently in a resource facility in which she can access the services she needs. She also attends mainstream school three days a week and therefore has sufficient ability to make her own decisions with regard to the relationships she engages in and to other areas of her life. In this sense, she is apt to make her own decisions, despite needing support to do so elsewhere. Even if she is deemed as having more difficulties making her own decision in certain areas, and final decisions must be made for her, she would still have to be respected. She expresses to Ruth that she loves her boyfriend, and Ruth therefore needs to respect Samantha's feelings.

Care

The word 'care', whether in terms of care plans, care management or simply social care, has different meanings in different contexts. This observation is echoed by Banks and Gallagher (2009), who assert that care as a virtue is difficult to define because there are so many meanings attached to the term. As such, we will propose a definition of care that stresses the characteristic of social workers involved in relationships with service users and that includes aspects of responsibility and concern. The notion of caring also involves emotions that affect the relationships between carers and persons cared for.

In the above case study, Ruth and Samantha have been working together for 18 months. As such, it is likely that their experience of care has changed during this period. At the beginning of the relationship, the notion of responsibility may have been devoid of emotions, more formal and probably more policy orientated. Furthermore, Ruth now acknowledges that Samantha tends to remind her of her own daughter. This has the potential of creating a range of emotions in the caring relationship. As the helping relationship developed, it may also have changed in nature and fostered a deeper relation of trust.

So what does 'caring' mean in this situation? Care, as a virtue, would cause Ruth to recognise her emotions while working with Samantha. Even despite her emotions, caring here would require Ruth to intervene with Samantha within the standards set out in the Code of Practice, that is, that no action or omission on her part should harm the well-being of service users (Scottish Social Services Council 2009:21). A caring relationship between Ruth and Samantha would therefore imply that Ruth take the appropriate means to ensure that Samantha is aware of the risk to which she may be exposing herself. Indeed, 'Difficulties in understanding and communication may mean that people with learning disabilities may be more susceptible to manipulation and exploitation and so vulnerable to certain kinds of crime and abuse' (Joint Committee on Human Rights 2008: 15). Moreover, Ruth should ensure that Samantha understands her right to be treated with dignity and respect as a human being.

Trustworthiness

Trustworthiness is a central quality of social work and is clearly recognised in each of the Council's codes of practice. In the case of Ruth's story, Samantha has trusted her social worker by confiding in her that her boyfriend was doing something when 'stressed' in her company. While it is not clear, in this case study, what is happening when Samantha and her boyfriend are together, Ruth has some concerns about Samantha being at risk of physical violence. When social workers engage in a relationship with a service user, they have a duty to explain the policy regarding confidentiality, as well as its limits, before anything is disclosed to the social worker. Therefore, Samantha should be aware that Ruth, as a social worker, should not disclose this information or any other information shared during the intervention to anyone else, except where there is clear evidence of serious risk to the service user or to others in the community. In these exceptional circumstances, social workers, on the basis of professional consideration and consultation, must limit any such breach of confidence to the needs of the situation at the time (BASW 2002: 10).

With regard to the case study, Ruth therefore must ask herself whether she considers this a serious threat to the service user and whether it warrants compromising her relationship with the service user. In this particular situation, it is clear that the service user may be exposed to some risk, but the social worker needs to ask herself about the seriousness of the risk involved. For example, because Samantha has discussed her private life with her social worker, she must feel, to a certain extent, that she has developed a relationship of trust with her. Otherwise, she may not feel the need to disclose personal information to her social worker. Simply put, this kind of disclosure about boyfriends is not what is usually expected as part of the social work services of an adult disability team. Therefore, a trustworthy social worker will make sure that she explains the limits of confidentiality to the service user at the beginning of the relationship and that she will remain open as to how she will perceive the situation. The social worker will want to reason based on the evidence she has regarding the situation and will carefully analyse its seriousness. In this case study, we can identify a presence of risk, but we must reason and deliberate as to whether the risk is imminent and serious enough to compromise the relationship with the service user by taking further action that directly involves her private life. In this particular case, and based on the perspectives of Virtue Ethics and the ethics of care, Ruth should continue to develop the relationship of trust with Samantha so that she can continue to share her concerns with her and support her in her decisions regarding the situation.

Justice

Much like for care, there are many ways of understanding the notion of 'justice'. For example, justice could be understood from a Rawslian or Utilitarian perspective (see Chapter 7), or as a Kantian principle of universality (see Chapter 6). While we are aware that there are many definitions and perspectives regarding justice, we shall understand justice in this chapter as being a virtue or character trait that allows a person to treat others equally and to promote a situation in which everyone can flourish and exercise their rights.

In this context, for Ruth to be a 'virtuous' social worker who embodies justice, she must, on the one hand, inform Samantha of her rights as a service user, and, on the other, hand treat Samantha within the perspective of human rights.

As to informing Samantha of her rights, the policy regarding learning disabilities in the four countries is clear:

> a commitment to enabling people with learning disabilities to live as equal citizens in the community alongside their non-disabled peers, with choice and control over their lives, and the support they need to enable this . . . and that *Valuing People* explicitly name that good services will help people with learning disabilities develop opportunities to form relationships, including ones of a physical and sexual nature (Joint Committee on Human Rights 2008).

Therefore, in acting with a sense of justice, Ruth will make sure that Samantha is aware of her rights and that these rights will be upheld during the intervention. In practical terms, this means that Ruth must support Samantha in understanding that, as a woman, she is free to choose with whom she engages in a relationship; at the same time, however, Samantha should be treated with respect in that relationship, despite her learning disability.

On the other hand, Ruth will also need to make sure that she treats Samantha with dignity and respect during the intervention. This echoes one of the principles of the ethical document of the International Federation of Social Workers:

> Respecting the right to self-determination – social workers should respect and promote people's right to make their own choices and decisions, irrespective of their values and life choices, provided this does not threaten the rights and legitimate interests of others (2005).

This means that Ruth must not treat Samantha differently because of her learning disability. If Samantha's relationship with her boyfriend becomes violent, Ruth should discuss with Samantha the different options and services available. Rather than taking unilateral action, Ruth should support Samantha in her own decision and help her look at the different possibilities of ending her relationship with her boyfriend.

Integrity

The BASW (2002) asserts that integrity comprises honesty, reliability, openness and impartiality, and is an essential value in the practice of social work. What does acting with integrity mean from a Virtue Ethics and ethics of care perspective in relation to Ruth's story?

Honesty means that Ruth should be open with Samantha and tell her that she is concerned about her safety. This was discussed more extensively above with regard to trustworthiness. Ruth should also make sure that she explores her own value base and ensure that her judgement is not clouded by personal values that she may hold which would affect her reading of the situation. This would help Ruth avoid placing her own beliefs before Samantha's needs and interests (BASW 2002, Principle 3.4.2 a). While it is unlikely that Ruth has any prejudices against people with disabilities since her own daughter has a long-term illness, behaving with integrity would also mean believing that everyone has the ability, when supported appropriately, to make decisions for themselves. Acting with integrity here would be to consider Samantha's needs and wishes about the situation, and although Samantha may express herself in a way that Ruth disagrees with, Ruth should not try to coerce Samantha into making a decision. The IFSW and IASSW (2004a) state that acting with integrity also includes not abusing the relationship of trust with service users, recognising the boundaries between personal and professional life and not abusing one's position for personal benefit or gain. In Samantha's situation, Ruth must act in such a manner as to recognise the limits between her personal and professional life, and because of the nature of the relationship, she must avoid treating Samantha like her own daughter, but as an adult needing services with regard to her disability. Ruth should also seek to discuss the situation with her supervisor and seek support if needed.

Criticality

Criticality is an important element of social work and is discussed in the National Occupational Standards for Social Work (2002) as a significant aspect of social work practice. Criticality, according to Adams *et al.* (2002: xxi), is the faculty that

> enables us to question the knowledge we have and our own involvement with clients, including our taken-for-granted understanding. It enables us to assess situations so as to make structural connections that penetrate the surface of what we encounter and locate what is apparent within wider contexts. Criticality therefore involves a process of reflection, an ability to reassess our own judgement and stresses a particular emphasises on the structural analysis of the situation we are observing or involved in.

To be critical in Samantha's situation, therefore, requires that Ruth examine her knowledge and explore it in relation to the work she is undertaking with the service user. For example, she may want to check that the relevant policy and theory she is using are indeed relevant to the situation; she should not simply apply guidelines that seem to fit in the first instance. She should explore, for example, best evidence regarding women who are victims of violence and the risks to which certain vulnerable groups may be more exposed. Being critical also means examining Samantha's situation using a more structural analysis and repositioning issues of gender, disabilities and socio-economic conditions central to this analysis and reasoning of the case. Is Samantha really at risk, or are Ruth's own prejudices affecting her professional judgement? Would it be possible that the marks on Samantha's arm have been caused by someone else? What policy is the agency trying to enforce? What is the supervisor's reading of the situation? What are the reasons behind the warden's telephone call? Are there any signs of disabilism? What is the view of the support health worker? Does he or she also have concerns about the situation? What, indeed, is Samantha's perception of the situation?

A critical social worker will take the time to think about how structural elements and issues of power that are identified can shape the analysis of the situation. Aspects of criticality as a virtue can also be found in the BASW (2002: 6–7) Code of Ethics under the umbrella term 'competence': social workers must

> reflect on the nature and source of social problems and on ways of addressing them; to contribute to promoting culturally appropriate practice and culturally sensitive services; and to identify, develop, use, and disseminate knowledge, theory, and skill for social work practice.

While the BASW notion of competence is broader than the one used by Adams *et al.* (2002), there are similarities such as the ability to analyse problems from a broader perspective through the use of theory and knowledge and to develop a type of practice that stresses the importance of non-oppressive values. These elements will provide social workers with a better understanding of the situations they face and allow them to form their own judgements regarding solutions.

Courage

The last virtue we wish to explore in relation to the above case study is 'courage'. Courage as a virtue has been considered important since ancient times and is still relevant to contemporary social work practice. Courage, according to Aristotle, can be developed first by being able to recognise situations that need to be changed, and secondly, by being able to stand our ground. We can therefore understand courage as a quality that, on the one hand, allows us to recognise practice that needs to be challenged and, on the other, gives us the strength of character to carry the decision forward, regardless of how difficult things may become.

In Ruth's story, the social worker must be able to recognise that Samantha reminds her of her own daughter and that this may affect her analysis of the situation and potentially cloud her judgement as to the best way to intervene. Furthermore, the social worker must be able to acknowledge the possible obstacles facing her should she decide to leave the situation as is, that is, supporting Samantha as an adult who is able to make her own decisions. The social worker will also have to take into consideration the course of action the organisation is endorsing and how this might affect her own course of action. For example, issues of risk management may have become dominant from the agency's point of view, and this may potentially affect Ruth's judgement in making her decision in ways that are not compatible with the virtues discussed above. As O'Brian (2003: 391) explains,

> professional judgment becomes circumscribed . . . the social worker's role is somewhat different than ones that are based on the two values of personal caring and social justice. A third value base appears to have emerged that we might call 'resource and risk management'.

As seen in the case study, Ruth is working for an organisation that wants her to intervene more directly in the case. A courageous social worker will take appropriate means to resist such pressure if her chosen course of action is to not follow the advice of her supervisor. Courage can therefore be an important virtue here, in that it may help the social worker carry her decision forward even as things become more difficult. Ethical issues of this type, that is, involving a conflict of loyalty between the user's interest and agency policy, has been identified by the IFSW and IASSW (2004a) as an important area for the emergence of ethical dilemmas and problems in practice. A courageous social worker will therefore have the strength to recognise possible conflicts and to carry through with the decision they have made despite the odds.

Professionalism in social work: the virtuous, caring social worker

The above virtues, as we have seen, are not always mutually exclusive and contain certain shared elements. For example, the theme of honesty was included in discussions about trustworthiness and integrity. This is a good example of how virtues are not exhibited alone and illustrates the need for developing them in sets. This is why, in a Virtue Ethics perspective, it is so important to develop a combination of different character traits. In the case study explored above, it is clear that Ruth could not have reached the best course of action based on a single virtue such as care. Instead, it is the combination of all the different virtues explored above that made Ruth position herself as a more ethical social worker. This demonstrates that ethics based on virtue must include a combination of character traits to be effective, and that no single virtue will lead to ethical social work practice.

As to which course of action would arise from Virtue Ethics and the ethics of care in this particular case, it is clear that Ruth may want to continue working with Samantha while respecting the latter's relationship with her boyfriend, as well as the decision she has made. Professionalism, in this sense, will require Ruth to continue monitoring the situation from a care perspective and critically analyse and re-evaluate it in light of new elements. She will also be aware of her own values and emotions and the impact they may have on her perception and analysis of the situation. She will respect Samantha in her choices and show compassion throughout. Even if the situation becomes difficult to manage and Ruth feels pressure from her agency to act in a particular way, she will have the courage and strength to persevere if she believes that it is the best way forward for Samantha and is compatible with the social work value base. More importantly, Ruth will continue to reason practically with regard to the situation as it unfolds and will remain flexible as her analysis of it evolves.

The virtuous social worker will then become habituated to reason and will exhibit the appropriate virtues necessary to maintain the best ethical social work practice at all times. This brings us to the conclusion of the chapter, in which we will briefly explore the application of Virtue Ethics and the ethics of care to modern social work practice.

Professionalism in context: the role of Virtue Ethics and the ethics of care in different organisations

We have seen throughout Chapters 3, 4 and 5 of this book, and as illustrated in Samantha's case study, the organisational work context can greatly impact on the way ethical practice is constructed, interpreted and maintained within social work. Indeed, the organisational work context often contributes to the development of relationships of power between the organisation and the social worker, and between the social worker, service users, groups and communities. In some situations, these relationships of power may result, for example, in the enactment of a particular legislation to protect a young person, or in limiting the application of a policy related to resource allocation, which may seriously affect preventative social work intervention for a particular service user.

How then can character-based ethics such as Virtue Ethics and the ethics of care help social workers in different organisational contexts? Some authors believe that a combination of Virtue Ethics and the ethics of care can help social workers operate ethically regardless of the work context. Indeed, MacIntyre (1999) asserts that cultivating virtues through practical reasoning is an effective mechanism for counteracting organisational contexts that may be detrimental to service users. If we truly understand what essentially constitutes a virtue, it becomes clear that practical reasoning can help social workers better identify their social work values and the nature of social work practice in general, without having to restrict themselves to the dominant forms of ethics seen in previous chapters, in which ethical principles are simply applied. Applying these principles without possessing the appropriate character traits or without having an awareness of the relationships in which we are involved can lead social workers to become technocrats instead of professionals capable of ethical judgement and reasoning.

MacIntyre points out that virtue is 'an acquired human quality' (1985: 191) rather than a feeling about rightness or wrongness. These personal qualities or virtues, when practised, will become part of the person instead of a one-off 'act of heroism' (Lynch and Lynch 2006). Understanding the primary concept of virtues and developing them through practical reasoning will help practitioners to feel more confident about their decisions and, consequently, to challenge, when necessary, the power relationships that exist in their organisational work context, between themselves and their employers and between themselves and service users. A note of caution, as MacIntyre (1985: 25) explains that Virtue Ethics is not always compatible with effectiveness and therefore does not always go hand in hand with the aims of organisations. To accomplish virtuous acts, social workers must exhibit many virtues at once; they must possess practical reasoning abilities in order to exhibit the right virtue at the right time and avoid succumbing to organisational pressure and bureaucracy. We acknowledge, however, that the impact of the organisational work context is significant for social workers and that challenging this context is not always an easy task.

Summary

We have explored in this chapter the major tenets of Virtue Ethics and the ethics of care, and how these perspectives can be relevant to modern social work practice. We have also seen that it is through practical reasoning that virtues can be developed and cultivated to the point that they become habits and integrated into all aspects of one's life. The ethics of care complements Virtue Ethics by emphasising the importance of the intervention relationship and the role of emotions in ethical reasoning. By examining Ruth's story, we observed how combining practical reason with the right character traits can help social workers act ethically and find the appropriate responses to ethical dilemmas in practice. Furthermore, by considering the application of various codes of ethics and conduct, we have seen how character-based ethics can use the various principles of social work practice and values to complement ethical reasoning as one of many ways to arrive at ethical decision making. We have also seen how certain virtues, such as courage and criticality, can help social workers challenge inappropriate use and abuse of power within organisations, and how these virtues can help social workers act ethically regardless of the context in which they practice.

Further reading

If you want to further your understanding of Virtue Ethics as applied to the helping profession, we recommend you read Banks, S. and Gallagher, A. (2009) *Ethics in the Professional Life,* Basingstoke, Palgrave-Macmillan. It provides a detailed account of different virtues that are needed in social and health professions and their application to practice.

Conclusion

True compassion is more than flinging a coin to a beggar. It comes to see that an edifice which produces beggars needs restructuring.

Martin Luther King, 4 April 1967, New York City

The challenges facing social work

Throughout this book we have been concerned to open up the ways in which social work students and practitioners can engage with ethical issues as they present in contemporary social work practice. Inevitably, this has led us into a discussion of many of the difficulties and challenges facing social work. The most significant of these is that we are now living through a major long-term economic crisis, which is accompanied by a new politics of austerity and further attacks on the vestiges of a welfare-based social contract. This impacts on social work practice very directly. First, the people who social workers work with are disproportionately from those sections of the community with the lowest incomes, the poorest educational outcomes, the poorest health outcomes and the highest levels of unemployment. In the present context social workers will continue to bear witness to increases in hardship for those people and communities, with all the attendant consequences this will have in terms of pressures on family relationships, multiple forms of social exclusion and criminalisation. Secondly, social work itself will be a victim of public expenditure cuts, meaning that the resources we have to assist people, both human and material, will be diminished. But perhaps the greatest threat to social work lies in the third point, which is about *the kind of social work* that will be practised in a period like this. In Part 1 of this book we examined aspects of social work's historic legacy, and one of the most important points we sought to express here was the idea that social work never has been and never will be just one thing – there have always been crucial value conflicts *within* social work; we characterised these as the 'two souls' of social work. As the chapters in Part 2 of the book seek to make clear, one of the most fundamental aspects of neo-liberal dominance in economics, politics and policy has been to change 'the meanings of welfare and the state as well as the policy and organizational structures to which they refer' (Clarke *et al.* 2000: 3). Many have wondered whether the present politics of austerity process places social work itself under threat. However, given the publics' demand for the authorities to 'do something' with regard to the social problems which catch public interest, and given the role social work plays in relation to these, it is probably the case that if social work was ever abolished it would need to be reinvented under another name. At the same time, one of the most significant impacts on social work in the present atmosphere of austerity and financial restrictions is, as we noted, about the kind of social work likely to be practised under these conditions. The riots that took place in the UK in summer 2011 are a worrying sign in the sense that the main governmental response was based on the idea that this behaviour was driven by 'pure criminality'; that those who took to the streets are simply people who have become morally debased. The idea that social inequality, exclusion and alienation, the existence of which is well documented (see, for example, Child Poverty Action Group 2011), form the context of the riots is not only dismissed, but in this discourse the very desire to understand the causes of this in a wider framework comes to be equated with condoning the worst aspects of the violence and antisocial behaviour that took place. At the level of social work we are already seeing the idea that this needs to be about being 'tough' with these people so that they 'understand the difference between right and wrong' (Jordan 2001). Unless social workers have the understandings that enable them to resist these dangerous oversimplifications, and the skills that enable them to work creatively with these individuals and communities, we see social work as an ethical enterprise being further undermined. It is for this reason that we see the reconstruction and strengthening of ideas of ethical practice in social work as so important.

The social worker as intellectual

In Chapter 1 of this book we discussed two different definitions of social work: one from the IFSW and one from Jacqui Smith, former UK Minister of Social Care. We noted that the IFSW definition represented the progressive and democratic impetus within social work, while Jacqui Smith's definition understood social workers' skills as practical *rather than* theoretical. Indeed it is interesting to note when one looks at the many different conceptualisations of social work, how this difference in understanding the social work role often focuses on whether social work is seen as a synthesis of the theoretical and the practical, as in the IFSW definition, or whether it represents the practical *as opposed to* the theoretical, as in Jacqui Smith's definition. Our argument is that if social workers are to make the link between an immediate presenting situation and its roots in the wider social structure, then this is about the engagement of the practitioner's conceptual and intellectual capacities. In an article which makes a definitive argument for social workers to see themselves as 'transformative intellectuals', Cowden and Singh argue that:

Central to reconstructing this sense of the social worker as a 'transformative intellectual' lies an understanding of the significance of the way social workers are witnesses to abuses of power and authority in society. The question of how social workers might respond to this is central to social work's 'praxis'; that is, the way it brings together the theoretical conceptual aspect of these situations with the practical tasks involved in attempting to deal with them (2009: 8).

To talk about 'social workers as intellectuals' is not to imply a coldly unemotional response to people's problems and difficulties, but it is to argue that sympathy is not enough in social work. The writer Oscar Wilde put this with characteristic wit when he argued 'the emotions of man [sic] are stirred much more easily than intelligence, and . . . it is much easier to have sympathy with suffering than with thought' (1973: 19). When we are confronted by the suffering of service users and their families that we see in practice, it is right that we respond emotionally, but not only so. True empathy and compassion come from the ability to theorise and thereby make sense of the issues that we see service users facing – and it is this intellectual understanding that forms a central tenet of social work's practical humanitarianism, as well being that which distinguishes social workers from being a good friend or a neighbour to the service user. It is therefore essential that we develop the ability to understand and name the wider structures and hidden assumptions which frame the conditions in which people live.

The social worker as practical reasoner

One of the concepts which links all the themes explored in the book together in a useful way is the concept of the 'practical reasoner'. We see a social worker committed to practical reasoning as someone who speaks with their own voice and is not simply, in Payne's phrase, 'travelling along guidelines and conventions' (Payne 2002: 126). A social worker committed to practical reasoning will be someone who looks beneath the surface – of course they must respond to immediate events, but they will also be situating these in a wider context, thinking beyond and through the immediate presenting situation. A social worker committed to practical reasoning will be someone who is prepared to think again and think differently, because a certain flexibility of understanding is at the essence of dealing with complex human problems, such as those involving loss, trauma or transition. But thinking differently does not mean simply thinking by yourself according to your own likes and dislikes.

Instead, practical reasoning which is achieved through critical awareness and refection must take place within what MacIntyre calls a 'practice' or a community of people sharing similar skills, values and ability. In other words, for ethical action to take place, the process must happen with other people who belong to the same practice community. This concept is very useful for social work, as we already have a community of practice that promotes practice standards and values, both internationally and locally, as shown in Chapter 2. The decisions a practical reasoner will take will be based on their practice values, and will take into consideration the historical legacy of the profession, as explored in Chapter 1. In the context of the argument developed in this book, this means that decisions taken by social workers in relation to ethical dilemmas should be actively informed by collectively agreed 'practice' or social work values. This leads us to pose the following question: how do we know that the social work or practice values are more important to promote than, say, organisational values promoted by the agencies for which you work for?

The work of Beauchamp (2001) is helpful in answering this question. He understands professional practice as involving a negotiation between both what he calls 'universal' and 'particular' morality (or practice principles). For Beauchamp 'universal morality' refers to the norms that are 'universally' agreed such as those found in internationally accepted charters, for example the human rights or, in the case of social work, the Social Work Statements of Principle (IFSW and IASSW 2004). The 'particular morality', on the other hand, is the 'universal moralities' that have been adapted to fit the local context. These particular norms utilise a universal justification, but in this approach universality does not mean uniformity; it is entirely justifiable to be able to take into consideration particular cultural, religious or institutional issues in a particular local context (Beauchamp 2001). In this sense, social work practice is based on a set of universal principles, but is also subject to principles which are derived from local contexts, which are those social workers deal with in their day-to-day work. Thierry de Duve makes a similar argument with regard to this negotiation between the universal, on one hand, and the local and particular, on the other:

> What is desirable is not primarily that we actually reach universal consensus, but that we defend the possibility for ourselves and others of making and communicating judgements of value, because by engaging in this activity we confirm our human commonality, the idea that we as humans, have a being in common (in Johnsson 2010: 123).

An approach like this points to the way social workers need to be able to negotiate the universal and the particular because as we have argued throughout the book, being able to take into consideration both levels of morality is linked to the exercise of practical reasoning skills.

Pullen-Sansfaçon (2011) elaborates this point when she discusses the way in which fostering professional values more deeply may help in ensuring a more ethical practice regardless of the practice setting or constraints. Indeed, she argues that 'because we know that core values and principles are central to the professional identity in social work (Asquith *et al.* 2005) and because internalised values mature into a coherent and dynamic set of ideas which guide belief and behaviour (Furnham and Ward 2001), we can assert that Social Workers would become better at resisting organisational constraints if they embedded fully the values of the profession in their own practice to the point that they become character traits or virtues' (Pullen-Sansfaçon 2011: 13). Many of the case studies we have used within this book have highlighted the distinction between the public expression of 'social work values' and our own personal values. The question of how much and of the way these are integrated will vary from person to person. However, the question of what this means is another dimension of the social worker as practical reasoner. Becoming a practical reasoner means that those values and dispositions become integral to the person, not only in professional practice. Consider, for example, a social work student or practitioner who considers themselves as committed to a concept of anti-oppressive practice while at work, but who remains silent during the weekend when racist or misogynist comments are made by friends or family. Becoming a practical reasoner is thus about always trying to integrate the values in which people believe in all aspects of their lives to the point where they become 'an acquired human quality' (MacIntyre 1985: 191). This also points to the links between practical reasoning and the importance of social workers valuing their intellectual capacities. Even if the change these offer appears small to begin with the process which is initiated can contribute to other broader changes in society.

And finally . . .

We have talked so far about the values of practical reasoning from the perspective of Virtue Ethics, which as we noted in Chapter 8, derive from the work of Aristotle and Ancient Greek philosophy. However, another crucial dimension of ethical thinking which we have also discussed in Chapters 3 and 6 is that of the Enlightenment, and the work of Immanuel Kant. One of Kant's works which is particularly useful for our concluding discussion are some of the comments he made in his final book, entitled *The Conflict of the Faculties* (1991). This is a book which concerns Kant's reflections on the French Revolution, but despite this specific context, Kant is posing broader questions which have considerable relevance for social work. A key question he is asking is whether, ethically speaking, there could ever be progress in human history. To use an example that we discussed in Chapter 1, did the abolition of child labour in the UK represent moral progress? One answer to this question is that un-equivocally did – it represented a major step forward for children's rights, for children's access to education and against the exploitation of the most vulnerable in the workplace. On the other hand, a less equivocal response might note that while it has been abolished in the wealthier more economically developed countries of Europe and the United States, it still continues in many poorer countries. Indeed a recent report in the *Guardian* newspaper (Ramesh 2007) details the way stone dug for patios, which have become popular in Britain in recent years, relies extensively on child labour from Rajasthan, India. Despite numerous attempts to draw attention to this, these reasonably priced products are very attractive to and popular with British homeowners. So who is right? Is the abolition of child labour in the UK something to be celebrated, or did it simply facilitate the end of that practice in one part of the world, allowing it to be shifted to another where children had even less power? Kant, who was thinking about the French Revolution at the time he wrote, accepted the complexity of the argument, and concluded that it was very hard to come down on one side or another of the argument as both were in their own way true. However, he also made the insightful point that while it is difficult to say whether a single event can ever be unequivocally a moment of freedom, what is most important are the signs which *point toward the possibility of freedom:*

> The recent Revolution of a people which is rich in spirit, may well either fail or succeed, accumulate misery or atrocity, it nevertheless arouses in the heart of all spectators (who are not themselves caught up in it) a taking of sides according to desires which borders on enthusiasm and which, since its very expression was not without danger, can only have been caused by the moral disposition of the human race (Kant 1991: 182).

What Kant is saying here is that the struggle against oppression and for a more just world involves a kind of enthusiasm here which is deeply moral, and it is this feeling which we need to hold onto regardless of the inevitably messy outcome of actual events. In this sense, the struggle against child labour by campaigners and the eventual impact that this had in legislation, on employment practices and on how we perceive children in society, was something which should be celebrated – it represented a moment that any person with a sense of morality and justice could relate to – even if the outcome has not gone as far as we would have hoped. By talking about Kant with his focus on intentionality we would not want to be seen here as suggesting that consequences do not matter – indeed not only would this be entirely wrong, but this would also obscure a wider truth, which is that all the moral frameworks we have discussed in this book have an inevitably partial approach. This does not have to mean that ethical theories are in competition with each other – it is rather that they are all cogs in a larger wheel. This could be seen to beg the question of how do we know which one to use in which situation? Our answer to this is twofold. First, it is essential to maintain one's focus on the universal morality or broader purpose of social work. Secondly that when it comes to making this choice we need to engage at all levels – mind, body and spirit.

Let us conclude with a recent example. In 2008 Barack Obama became the first ever black presidential candidate to win an election in the United States;

and this is a moment that both of us remembered with great clarity. While we were both totally aware of his limitations, his failures to stand up to the corporate elite and the military, and worrying absence of concrete details of how change was actually going to occur within his soaring rhetoric, nonetheless this was a profoundly emotional moment, and we described having tears in our eyes as we explained what this meant to our children. For all the ways in which we knew the hopes millions had invested in him were likely to be compromised, it was a moment in which we glimpsed a sign of freedom, and we felt this in our very being. It is in this spirit that we remain optimistic about the possibilities for genuine ethical and emancipatory practice within social work. For all the destructive forces which beset social workers in their attempts to make a difference, for all the way in which social work is compromised by bureaucracy and managerialism, the ethical impulse which animates the best elements in social work remain things that are worth believing in and fighting against the odds to make a reality.

References

Adams, R. (2003) *Social Work and Empowerment.* BASW/Palgrave Macmillan, London.

Adams, R. (2008) *Empowerment, Participation and Social Work.* BASW/Palgrave Macmillan, London.

Adams, R., Dominelli, L. and Payne, M. (2002) *Critical Practice in Social Work.* Palgrave, Basingstoke.

Albo, G. (2007) 'Neoliberalism and Discontent'. In Panitch, L., and Leys, C. (eds.) *The Socialist Register 2008*, pp. 354–62, Merlin Press, London.

Allen, C. (2007) *Housing Market Renewal and Social Class.* Routledge, London.

Almond, B. (1985) *Introducing Applied Ethics.* Blackwell, Oxford.

American Psychiatric Publishing (2010) *DSM-IV-TR- Diagnostic and Statistical Manual of Mental Disorders.* http://www.psychiatryonline.com/resourceTOC.aspx?resourceID=1, accessed 21 December 2010.

Aristotle (1999) *Nicomachean Ethics,* translated by W. D. Ross. Batoche Books, Kitchener.

Asquith, S., Clark, C. and Waterhouse, L. (2005) *The Role of the Social Worker in the 21st Century: A Literature Review.* Scottish Executive, Edinburgh.

Bailey, R. and Brake, M. (1975) *Radical Social Work.* Hodder & Stoughton, London.

Baistow, K. (1994) 'Liberation and Regulation? Some Paradoxes of Empowerment'. *Critical Social Policy* 14 (42), No. 3 Winter 94/95, 34–6.

Banks, S. (1995) *Ethics and Values in Social Work.* Macmillan, Basingstoke.

Banks, S. (2006) *Ethics and Values in Social Work,* 3rd edn. Palgrave-Macmillan, Basingstoke.

Banks, S. and Gallagher, A. (2009) *Ethics in the Professional Life.* Palgrave-Macmillan, Basingstoke.

Banks, S. and Williams, R. (2005) 'Accounting for Ethical Difficulties in Social Welfare Work: Issues, Problems and Dilemmas'. *British Journal of Social Work* 35, 1005–22.

Bar-On, A. (2002) 'Restoring Power to Social Work Practice'. *British Journal of Social Work* 32 (8), 997–1014.

BBC News (2010) *Bureaucracy Hampers Social Workers Survey Says. 28 July,* http://www.bbc.co.uk/news/education-10788737, accessed 30 March 2011.

Beckett, C. and Maynard, A. (2005) *Values and Ethics in Social Work.* Sage, London.

Beauchamp, T. (2001) 'Internal and External Standards for Medical Morality'. *Journal of Medicine and Philosophy* 26 (6), 601–19.

Beauchamp, T. L. and Childress, J. F. (2001) *Principles of Biomedical Ethics,* 5th edn. Oxford University Press, New York.

Biestek, F. (1961) *The Casework Relationship.* George Allen and Unwin, London.

Boland, K. (2006) 'Ethical Decision Making among Hospital Social Workers'. *Journal of Social Work Values and Ethics.* 3 (1), http://www.socialworker.com/jswve/content/view/27/44/, accessed 1 November 2010.

Bouquet, B. (2004) *Ethique et Travail Social.* Dunod, Paris.

Bourdieu, P. *et al.* (2002) *The Weight of the World: Social Suffering in Contemporary Society.* Polity Press, Cambridge.

Bowie, A. (2003) *Introduction to German Philosophy: From Kant to Habermas.* Polity Press, Cambridge.

British Association of Social Workers (2002) *Code of Ethics*. BASW, Birmingham.

Brown, K. and Rutter, L. (2006) *Critical Thinking for Social Work*. Learning Matters, Exeter.

Butler, I. and Drakeford, M. (2003) *Scandal, Social Policy and Social Welfare*. Policy Press, Bristol.

Callinicos, A. (2010) 'Two Cheers for Enlightenment Universalism: Or, Why It's Hard to Be an Aristotelian Revolutionary'. In Paul, B., and Kelvin, K. (eds.) *Virtue and Politics*, University of Notre Dame Press, Notre Dame.

Carey, M. (2008a) 'Everything Must Go? The Privatisation of State Social Work'. *British Journal of Social Work* 38 (5), 918–35.

Carey, M. (2008b) 'The Quasi-market Revolution in the Head: Ideology, Discourse, Care Management'. *Journal of Social Work* 8 (4), 341–62.

Case Con Manifesto. http://www.radical.org.uk/barefoot/casecon.htm, accessed August 2009.

Centre for Contemporary Cultural Studies (1982) *The Empire Strikes Back: Race and Racism in the 70's Britain*. Hutchinson, London.

Child Poverty Action Group (2011a) *Poverty: The Facts*. http://www.cpag.org.uk/povertyfacts/, accessed July 2011.

Child Poverty Action Group (2011b) *The Cuts: What They Mean for Families at Risk of Poverty*. http://www.cpag.org.uk/, accessed July 2011.

Clark, C. (2000) *Social Work Ethics: Politics, Principles and Practice*. Macmillan, Basingstoke.

Clark, C. (2005) 'The Deprofessionalisation Thesis, Accountability and Professional Character'. *Social Work and Society* 3 (2).

Clark, C. (2006) 'Moral Character in Social Work'. *British Journal of Social Work* 36, 75–89.

Clarke, J. (2000) *New Managerialism, New Welfare*. Sage, London.

Clarke, J. (2005) 'New Labour's Citizens; Activated, Empowered, Responsibilised, Abandoned'. *Critical Social Policy* 25 (4), 447–63.

Clifford, D. and Burke, B. (2009) *Anti-oppressive Ethics and Values in Social Work*. Palgrave-Macmillan, Basingstoke.

Coard, B. (2005) 'How the West Indian Child I Made Educationally Sub-normal'. In Richardson, B. (ed.) *Tell I Like Is: How Our Schools Fail Black Children*, pp. 27–59, Boomarks Publications, London.

Collins, P. H. (2000) *Black Feminist Thought: Knowledge, Consciousness and the Politics of Empowerment*. Routledge, London.

Conference of Socialist Economists (CSE) (1980) *In and Against the State*. Pluto Press, London.

Conway, J. K. (ed.) (1992) *Written by Herself: Autobiographies of American Women*. Vintage Books, London.

Cowden, S. and Singh, G. (2006) 'The 'User': Friend, Foe or Fetish? A Critical Exploration of User Involvement in Health and Social Care. *Critical Social Policy* 27 (1), 5–23 Trouvé 2007.

Cowden, S. and Singh, G. (2009) 'Social Workers as Intellectuals: Reclaiming a Critical Praxis'. *European Journal of Social Work* 12 (4), 479–93.

Craib, I. (1997) *Classical Social Theory*. Oxford University Press, Oxford.

Crocker, R. H. (1992) *Social Work and Social Order: The Settlement Movement in Two Industrial Cities*. University of Illinois Press, Chicago.

Cruikshank, B. (1999) *The Will to Empower*. Cornell University Press, Ithaca and London.

Dale, H. (1998) 'Child Labour under Capitalism [1908]'. In Alexander, S. (ed.) *Women's Fabian Tracts*, pp. 53–72, Routledge, London.

De Beauvoir, S. (1972) *The Second Sex*. Pengiun Books Australia, Melbourne.

Department of Health (1998) *Fundamental Review of the CCETSW*. http://www.open. gov.uk/hdg1551.htm, accessed 10 November 1999.

Dixon, T. (2008) *The Invention of Altruism: Making Moral Meanings in Victorian Britain*. British Academy, London.

Dominelli, L. (2009) *Introducing Social Work*. Polity Press, Cambridge.

Doyle, Z. O., Miller, S. E. and Mirza, F. Y. (2009) 'Ethical Decision-making in Social Work: Exploring Personal and Professional Values'. *The Journal of Social Work Values and Ethics* 6 (1), online http://www.socialworker.com/jswve/content/view/113/67/, accessed 1 November 2010.

Du Gay, P. (2000) *In Praise of Bureaucracy: Weber – Organization – Ethics*. Sage, London.

Else, D. E. (2006) 'Oppression, Prejudice and Discrimination'. In Morrow, D. F., and Messinger, L. (eds.) *Sexual Orientation and Gender Expression in Social Work Practice*, pp. 43–80, Columbia University Press, New York.

Fanon, F. (1967) *Black Skins, White Masks*. Pluto Press, London.

Feather, N. T. (1992). Values, valences, expectations, and actions. *Journal of Social Issues*, 48, 109–124.

Ferguson, I. and Lavalette, M. (2007) 'The Social Worker as Agitator: The Radical Kernel of British Social Work'. In Lavalette, M. and Ferguson, I. *International Social Work and the Radical Tradition*, BASW, Birmingham.

Ferguson, I. and Lavalette, M. (2009) *Social Work after Baby P: Issues, Debates and Alternative Perspectives*. Liverpool Hope Press, Liverpool.

Fives, A. (2008) *Political and Philosophical Debates in Welfare*. Palgrave Press, Harmondsworth.

Foucault, M. (1967) *Madness and Civilisation*. Tavistock Publications, London.

Foucault, M. (1977) *Discipline and Punish*. Penguin Press, Harmondsworth.

Freire, P. (1972) *Pedagogy of the Oppressed*. Penguin, Harmondsworth.

Freire, P. (1990) *Interview with Carlos Torres*. http://aurora.icaap.org/talks/freire.html, accessed 23 November 2010.

Furnham, A. and Ward, C. (2001) 'Internalizing Values and Virtues'. In Columbus, F. (ed.) *Advances in Psychology Research*, pp. 229–54, Nova Science Publishers, New York.

Ghosh, S. (2009) *Sexuality, gender identity*. Emedecine. Last updated 19 May 2009. http:// emedicine.medscape.com/article/917990-overview, accessed 16 December 2010.

Giddens, A. (1998) *The Third Way*. Polity Press, Cambridge.

Gilligan, C. (1982) *A Different Voice*. Harvard University Press, Cambridge.

Graham, G. (2004) *Eight Theories of Ethics*. Routledge, London.

Griffiths, J. (2010) 'Children's Services Must House 18-year-old Asylum Seekers'. *Community Care*. 15 October 2010.

GSCC (General Social Care Council) (2002a) *Code of Practice for Social Care Workers*.

GSCC (General Social Care Council) (2002b) *FAQs about Us*. http://www.gscc.org.uk/gscc/ Templates/Anchor.aspx?NRMODE=Published&NRORIGINALURL=%2fAbout%2bus%2fF AQs%2babout%2bus%2f&NRNODEGUID=%7b38736449-DFE9-4709- B8AC-45E9F019E5D0%7d&NRCACHEHINT=NoModifyGuest#2, accessed 6 October 2005.

GSCC (General Social Care Council) (2010) *Code of Practice for Social Care Workers*. http://www.gscc.org.uk/cmsFiles/Registration/Codes%20of%20Practice/Codesof PracticeforSocialCareWorkers.pdf, accessed 5 May 2011.

GSCC (General Social Care Council) (no date) *Conduct*. http://www.gscc.org.uk/Conduct/, last accessed 9 November 2010, GSCC, London.

Guardian (2011) Jarvis to escape prosecution over Potters Bar crash. 17 March 2011.

Hall, S. (2007) 'Universities, Intellectuals, Multitudes——An Interview with Stuart Hall'. In Cote, M., Day, R. J. F., and de Peuter, G. (eds) *Utopian Pedagogy: Radical Experiments against Neoliberal Globalization*, pp. 108–128, University of Toronto Press, Toronto.

Halwani, R. (2003) Care ethics and virtue ethics. *Hypatia* 18 (3), 161–92.

Harrington, D. and Dolgoff, R. (2008) 'Hierarchies of Ethical Principles for Ethical Decision Making in Social Work'. *Ethics and Social Welfare* 2 (2), 183–96.

Harris, J. (1999) 'State Social Work and Social Citizenship in Britain: From Clientilism to Consumerism'. *British Journal of Social Work* 29 (6), 915–37.

Harvey, D. (2007) *A Brief History of Neo-liberalism*. Oxford University Press, Oxford and London.

Harvey, D. Interviewed by Sasha Lilley about neo-liberalism. http://www.indybay.org/newsitems/2009/03/09/18575771.php, accessed 19 August 2010.

Hicks, S. (2008) 'Thinking through Sexuality'. *Journal of Social Work* 8 (1), 65–82.

Hindess, B. (1996) *Discourses of Power: From Hobbes to Foucault*. Blackwell, Oxford.

Hochschild, A. (1989) *The Second Shift*. Penguin Books, Harmondsworth.

Hooker, R. (1996) *Women during the European Enlightenment*. http://www.wsu.edu/~dee/ENLIGHT/WOMEN.HTM, accessed 8 February 2010.

Horner, N. (2003) *What Is Social Work? Context and Perspectives*. Learning Matters, Essex.

Houlgate, S. (2005) *Introduction to Hegel: Freedom, Truth and History*. Blackwell, Oxford.

Houston, S. (2003) 'Establishing the Virtue in Social Work: A Response to McBeath and Webb'. *British Journal of Social Work* 33, 819–24.

Hugman, R. (2005) *New Approaches in Ethics for the Caring Profession*. Palgrave-Macmillan, Basingstoke.

IFSW and IASSW (2004a) *Global Standards for the Education and the Training of the Social Work Profession*. Adelaide, Australia. http://www.ifsw.org/cm_data/GlobalSocialWork Standards2005.pdf, accessed 11 September 2009.

IFSW and IASSW (2004b) *Ethics in Social Work, Statement of Principles*. Online. http://www.ifsw.org/f38000032.html, last accessed 27 October 2011.

International Federation of Social Workers (2000) *Ethics in Social Work, Statement of Principles*. http://www.ifsw.org/f38000032.html, last accessed 18 November 2010.

International Federation of Social Workers (2010) *Human Rights* website. http://www.ifsw.org/p38001792.html#el38005151, accessed 29 April 2011.

Jaggar, A. M. (2000) 'Feminist Ethics'. In Lafolette, H. (ed.) *The Blackwell Guide to Ethical Theory*, pp. 348–74, Blackwell, Oxford.

James, C. L. R. (1963) *The Black Jacobins*. Penguin, London.

Johnsson, S. (2010) 'The Ideology of Universalism'. *New Left Review* 63 (May/June), 115–26.

Joint Committee on Human Rights (2008) *A Life Like Any Other? Human Rights and Adults with Learning Disabilities. Seventh Report 2007–2008 Volume 1*. House of Commons, London, The Stationery Office Limited. http://www.publications.parliament.uk/pa/jt200708/jtselect/jtrights/40/4005.htm, last viewed 26 February 2010.

Jones, C. (1998) 'Social Work and Society'. In Dominelli *et al. Social Work: Themes, Issues and Critical Debates*, pp. 41–9. Palgrave, Basingstoke.

Jones, G. S. (1976) *Outcast London: A Study in the Relationship between Classes in Victorian Society*. Penguin, Harmondsworth.

Jordan, B. (2001) 'Tough Love: Social Work, Social Exclusion and the Third Way'. *British Journal of Social Work* 31 (4), 527–46.

Jordan, B. (2004) 'Emancipatory Social Work? Opportunity or Oxymoron'? *British Journal of Social Work* 34 (1), 5–19.

Kant, I. (1785) *Groundwork of the Metaphysics of Morals*. http://www.justiceharvard.org/resources/immanuel-kant-groundwork-for-the-metaphysics-of-morals-1785/, accessed 19 August 2011.

Kant, I. (1991) 'The Conflict of Faculties'. In *Political Writings*, pp. 176–7, Cambridge University Press, Cambridge.

Karacaer, S., Gohar, R., Aygun, M. and Sayin, C. (2009) 'Effects of Personal Values on Auditor's Ethical Decisions'. *Journal of Business Ethics* 88 (1), 53–64.

Kennedy, N. and Hellen, M. (2010) 'Gender Variant Children: More than a Theoretical Challenge'. *Graduate Journal of Social Sciences* 7 (2), 25–43.

Kinner, R. T., Kernes, J. L. and Dautheribes, T. M. (2000) 'A Short List of Universal Moral Values'. *Counselling and Values* 45, 4–16.

Knapp, P. and Spector, A. (2011) *Crisis and Change Today: Basic Questions of Marxist Sociology*. Rowan and Littlefield, Maryland and Plymouth.

Kohli, R. K. S. and Mitchell, F. (eds.) (2007) *Working with Unaccompanied Asylum Seeking Children: Issues for Policy and Practice*. Palgrave Macmillan, London.

Kosciw, J. G., Diaz, E. and Greytak, E. (2007) *National School Climate Survey: The Experiences of Lesbian, Gay, Bisexual and Transgender Youth in our Nation's Schools*. GLSEN, New York.

Lamont, C. and Favor, C. (2007) *Distributive Justice. Stanford Encyclopedia of Philosophy*. http://plato.stanford.edu/entries/justice-distributive/. First published 22 September 1996; substantive revision 5 March 2007, accessed 12 August 2011.

Langan, M. (1998) 'Radical Social Work'. In Dominelli *et al. Social Work: Themes, Issues and Critical Debates*, pp. 209–17. Palgrave, Basingstoke.

Langer S. and Martin, J. I. (2004) 'How Dresses Can Make You Mentally Ill: Examining Gender Identity Disorder in Children'. *Child and Adolescent Social Work Journal* 21 (1), 5–23.

Lavalette, M. and Ferguson, I. (2007) *International Social Work and the Radical Tradition*, pp. 11–31, Venture Press, Birmingham.

Legault, G. A. (1999) *Professionalisme et Deliberation Ethique*. Presse de l'Université du Québec.

Lewis, G. (1998) 'Coming Apart at the Seams: The Crisis of the Welfare State. In Hughes, G., and Lewis, G., *Unsettling Welfare: The Reconstruction of Social Policy*, pp. 39–80, Routledge, Open University, London.

Lipsky, M. (1980) *Street Level Bureaucracy: Dilemmas of the Individual in Public Service*. Russell Sage Foundation, New York.

Lukes, S. (1974) *Power: A Radical View*. Macmillan, London.

Lynch, D. T. and Lynch, C. E. (2006) 'Aristotle, MacIntyre and Virtue Ethics'. *Public Administration and Public Policy* 116, 55–74.

MacIntyre, A. (1985) *After Virtue*, 2nd edn. Duckworth, London.

MacIntyre, A. (1999) *Rational Dependent Animals*. Duckworth, London.

Marshall, G. (ed.) (1998) *Dictionary of Sociology*, 2nd edn. Oxford University Press, Oxford.

Marx, K. (1848) *The Communist Manifesto*. Verso, London, 1998.

Marx, K. (1975a) 'Critique of Hegel's Philosophy of Right'. In Marx, K. (ed.) *Early Writings*, pp. 57–198, Penguin, Harmondsworth.

Marx, K. (1975b) 'Theses on Feuerbach'. In Coletti, L. (ed.) *Marx: Early Writings*, pp. 421–3, Pelican Marx Library/New Left Review Editions, Penguin Books, Harmondsworth.

Mayhew, H. (1968) *London Labour and the London Poor*, with a new introduction by John D. Rosenberg. Dover Publications, New York. First Published 1851.

McBeath, G. and Webb, S. (2002) Virtue Ethics and Social Work: Being Lucky, Realistic, and Not Doing One's Duty'. *British Journal of Social Work* 25, 423–39.

McLaren, P. and Da Silva, T. (1993) 'Decentring Pedagogy: Critical Literacy, Resistance and Politics of Memory'. In *Paulo Freire: A Critical Encounter*, Routledge, London.

Mill, J. S. (2004) *Utilitarianism (1863 edition)*. Parker Son and Bourn, London.

Mill, J. S. (1989) *On Liberty and Other Essays*. Cambridge University Press, Cambridge.

Morse, J. (1999) 'The Missing Link between Virtue Theory and Business Ethics'. *Journal of Applied Philosophy* 16 (1), 47–58.

Moss, B. (2007) *Values*. Russell House Publishing, Lyme Regis.

Mullaly, B. (2002) *Challenging Oppression: A Critical Social Work Approach*. Oxford University Press, Ontario.

Mullaly, B. (2010) *Challenging Oppression and Confronting Privilege*, 2nd edn. Oxford University Press, Ontario.

Mullender, A. and Ward, D. (1991a) *Self-Directed Groupwork: Users Take Action for Empowerment*. Withing and Birch, London.

Mullender, A. and Ward, D. (1991b) 'Empowerment and Oppression: An Indissoluble Pairing for Contemporary Social Work'. *Critical Social Policy* 11.

Munro, E. (2011) *Munro Review of Child Protection: Interim Report*. http://www.education.gov.uk/munroreview/downloads/Munrointerimreport.pdf, accessed 16 May 2011.

National Institute for Social Work (1982) *Social Workers, Their Roles and Tasks (Barclay Committee)*. Oxford Square Press, London.

O'Brian, C. (2003) 'Resource and Educational Empowerment: A Social Work Paradigm for the Disenfranchised'. *Research in Social Work* 13 (3), 388–99.

OFSTED (2010) *Safeguarding and Looked After Children: National Results for Children's Social Work Practitioners Survey 2010 (NAT '10)*. OFSTED, Manchester.

O'Sullivan, T. (1999) *Decision Making in Social Work*. Palgrave, Basingstoke.

Pakizeh, A., Gebauer, J. E. and Maio, G. R. (2007) 'Basic Human Values: Inter-value Structure in Memory'. *Journal of Experimental Social Psychology* 43 (2007), 458–65.

Pampel, F. C. (2000) *Sociological Lives and Ideas: An Introduction to the Classical Theorists*. Macmillan, Basingstoke.

Parker, M. (2002) *Against Management*. Polity Press, Cambridge.

Parkin, F. (2002) *Max Weber (Routledge Key Sociologists)*. Routledge, London.

Payne, M. (2002) 'Social Work Theory and Reflective Practice'. In Adams *et al.* (2002) (2nd edn.) *Social Work Themes, Issues and Critical Debates*, pp. 123–139, Palgrave, Basingstoke.

Payne, M. (2005) *The Origins of Social Work*. Palgrave Macmillan, Basingstoke.

Petrie, S. (2009) 'Are the International and National Codes of Ethics for Social Work in the UK as Useful as a Chocolate Teapot'? *Journal of Social Work Values and Ethics* 6, 2.

Pirsig, R. (1999) *Zen and the Art of Motorcycle Maintenance: An Enquiry in Values*. Vintage Press, New York.

Polyani, K. (2001) *The Great Transformation*. Beacon Press, Boston.

Porter, R. (1990) *The Enlightenment*. Macmillan, Basingstoke.

Powell, F. (2001) *The Politics of Social Work*. Sage, London.

Pullen-Sansfaçon, A. (2011) 'Ethics and Conduct in Self-directed Groupwork: Some Lessons for the Development of a More Ethical Social Work Practice'. *Ethics and Social Welfare* Vol 5. Issue 4 (2011) pp 361–379.

Rachels, J. (1986) *The Elements of Moral Philosophy*. Random House, New York.

Ramazanoglu, C. and Holland, J. (2002) *Feminist Methodology: Challenges and Choices*. Sage Publications, London.

Ramesh, R. (2007) *Between a Rock and a Hard Place – How UK Patios Rely on Child Labour*. *The Guardian*, 13 February 2007. http://www.guardian.co.uk/world/2007/feb/13/india.randeepramesh, accessed 28 July 2011.

Rawls, J. (1971) *A Theory of Justice*. Harvard University Press, Cambridge.

Reamer, F. (1982) *Ethical Dilemmas in Social Services*. Columbia University Press, New York.

Revans, L. (2007) *Bureaucracy: Social Workers Bogged Down by Paperwork. Community Care.* 26 April, http://www.communitycare.co.uk/Articles/2007/04/26/104274/Bureaucracy-social-workers-bogged-down-by-paperwork.-Exclusive.htm, accessed 30 March 2011.

Rhodes, M. (1986) *Ethical Dilemmas in Social Work Practice*. Family Service America Press, Milwaukee, Wisconsin[8361].

Ricoeur, P. (1985) in Bouquet, B. (2004) *Éthique et Travail Social*. Dunod, Paris.

Ricoeur, P. (1990) *Soi même comme un autre*: Seuil, Paris.

Rojek, C., Peacock, G. and Collins, S. (1988) *Social Work and Received Ideas*. Routledge, London.

Rousseau, J. (1988) *The Social Contract*. Wordsworth Classics, Hertfordshire.

Said, E. (1978) *Orientalism*. Penguin Books, Harmondsworth.

Schwartz, S. H. (1992) 'Universals in the Content and Structure of Values: Theoretical Advances and Empirical Tests in 20 countries'. In Zanna, M. (ed.) *Advances in Experimental Social Psychology,* pp. 1–65, Academic Press, San Diego.

Scottish Social Services Council (2009) *Codes of Practice for Social Services Workers and Employers*. Scottish Social Services Council, Dundee.

Simmonds, J. and Merredew, F. (2010) *The Health Needs of Unaccompanied Asylum Seeking Children and Young People EP23–LAC 9.4 Unaccompanied asylum seeking children,* pp. 1–6. BAAF, London.

Smart, B. (2003) 'Michel Foucault'. In Ritzer, G. (ed.) *The Blackwell Companion to Major Contemporary Social Theorists,* Blackwell, Oxford.

Smith, R. (2008) *Social Work and Power*. Palgrave Macmillan, Basingstoke.

Jones, Ferguson, Lavalette and Penketh. (2006) Social Work Manifesto http://www.socialworkfuture.org/index.php/swan-organisation/manifesto, accessed 26 May 2011.

Strom-Gottfried, K. and D'aprix, A. (2006) 'Ethics for Academics'. *Social Work Education* 25 (3), 225–44.

Sysneros *et al.* (2008) in Mullaly (2010) *Challenging Oppression and Confronting Privilege*. Oxford University Press, Canada.

Thane, P. (1982) *Foundations of the Welfare State*. Longman, London.

Townsend, Mrs (1998) 'The Case against the Charity Organisation Society [1911]'. In Alexander, S. (ed.) *Women's Fabian Tracts,* pp. 179–99, Routledge, London.

Turner, B. (1996) *For Weber: Essays on the Sociology of Fate*. Sage Publications, London.

United Nations (1948) *The Universal Declaration of Human Rights*. http://www.un.org/en/documents/udhr/index.shtml, accessed 19 August 2011.

Vardy, P. and Grosch, P. (1999) *The Puzzle of Ethics*, 2nd edn. HarperCollins, London.

Wade, J., Mitchell, F. and Baylis, G. (2005) *Unaccompanied Asylum Seeking Children: The Response of Social Work Services*. BAAF, London.

Wall, G. B. (1974) *Introduction to Ethics*. Charles E Merril Publishing Company, Ohio.

Wallace, R. J. (2003) *Practical Reason. Stanford Encyclopedia of Philosophy*. Online http://plato.stanford.edu/entries/practical-reason/, last accessed 27 october 2011.

Warburton, N. (1999) *Philosophy: The Basics*. Routledge, New York.

Weber, M. (2005) 'On the Difficulty of Destroying the Bureaucracy'. In Kahlberg, S. (ed.) *Max Weber,* pp. 214–16, Blackwell, Oxford.

Weinberg, M. (2008) Structural social work: A moral compass for ethics in practice. *Critical Social Work* 9 (1).

West, C. (1999) *The Cornell West Reader*. Basic Civitas Books, New York.

Wilde, O. (1973) 'The Soul of Man under Socialism'. In *De Profundis and Other Writings,* pp. 17–54, Penguin, Harmondsworth.

Witkin, S. L. (2000) 'Ethics-R-Us'. *Social Work* 45 (3), 197–200.

Woodrofe, K. (1962) *From Charity to Social Work*. Routledge Kegan Paul, London.

Woolstonecraft, M. (2007) *A Vindication of the Rights of Woman*. Pearson Longman, London and New York.

Zippay, A. (1995) 'The Politics of Empowerment'. *Social Work* 40 (2), 263–7.

Žižek, S. (2009a) *Violence*. Profile Books, London.

Žižek, S. (2009b) *First as Tragedy, Then as Farce*. Verso, London.

Index